Telemedicine in the ICU

Editors

RICHARD W. CARLSON
COREY SCURLOCK

CRITICAL CARE CLINICS

www.criticalcare.theclinics.com

Consulting Editor
RICHARD W. CARLSON

April 2015 • Volume 31 • Number 2

ELSEVIER

1600 John F. Kennedy Boulevard • Suite 1800 • Philadelphia, Pennsylvania, 19103-2899

http://www.theclinics.com

CRITICAL CARE CLINICS Volume 31, Number 2
April 2015 ISSN 0749-0704, ISBN-13: 978-0-323-35971-9

Editor: Patrick Manley
Developmental Editor: Casey Jackson

Critical Care Clinics (ISSN: 0749-0704) is published quarterly by Elsevier Inc., 360 Park Avenue South, New York, NY 10010-1710. Months of issue are January, April, July, and October. Business and Editorial Offices: 1600 John F. Kennedy Blvd., Suite 1800, Philadelphia, PA 19103-2899. Customer Service Office: 6277 Sea Harbor Drive, Orlando, FL 32887-4800. Periodicals postage paid at New York, NY and additional mailing offices. Subscription prices are $210.00 per year for US individuals, $503.00 per year for US institution, $100.00 per year for US students and residents, $255.00 per year for Canadian individuals, $630.00 per year for Canadian institutions, $300.00 per year for international individuals, $630.00 per year for international institutions and $150.00 per year for Canadian and foreign students/residents. To receive student/resident rate, orders must be accompanied by name of affiliated institution, date of term, and the signature of program/residency coordinator on institution letterhead. Orders will be billed at individual rate until proof of status is received. Foreign air speed delivery is included in all *Clinics* subscription prices. All prices are subject to change without notice. POSTMASTER: Send address changes to *Critical Care Clinics*, Elsevier Periodicals Customer Service, 11830 Westline Industrial Drive, St. Louis, MO 63146. **Customer Service: 1-800-654-2452 (US). From outside of the US, call 1-314-447-8871. Fax: 1-314-447-8029. E-mail: journalscustomerservice-usa@ elsevier.com (for print support) or journalsonlinesupport-usa@elsevier.com (for online support).**

Reprints. For copies of 100 or more of articles in this publication, please contact the Commercial Reprints Department, Elsevier Inc., 360 Park Avenue South, New York, NY 10010-1710. Tel.: 212-633-3874; Fax: 212-633-3820; E-mail: reprints@elsevier.com.

Critical Care Clinics is also published in Spanish by Editorial Inter-Medica, Junin 917, 1er A, 1113, Buenos Aires, Argentina.

Critical Care Clinics is covered in *MEDLINE/PubMed (Index Medicus), EMBASE/Excerpta Medica, Current Concepts/Clinical Medicine, ISI/BIOMED,* and *Chemical Abstracts.*

Contributors

CONSULTING EDITOR

RICHARD W. CARLSON, MD, PhD
Staff, Medical Intensive Care Unit, Maricopa Medical Center; Professor, College of
Medicine, Mayo Clinic, Phoenix, Arizona; Professor, University of Arizona College of
Medicine, Scottsdale, Arizona

EDITORS

RICHARD W. CARLSON, MD, PhD
Staff, Medical Intensive Care Unit, Maricopa Medical Center; Professor, College of
Medicine, Mayo Clinic, Phoenix, Arizona; Professor, University of Arizona College of
Medicine, Scottsdale, Arizona

COREY SCURLOCK, MD, MBA
National Medical Director, Advanced ICU Care, New York, New York

AUTHORS

OMAR BADAWI, PharmD, MPH
Senior Clinical Scientist, Hospital to Home, Philips Healthcare; Adjunct Assistant
Professor, Department of Pharmacy Practice and Science, University of Maryland
School of Pharmacy, Baltimore, Maryland

JOSEPH J. BANDER, MD
Director of Surgical Intensive Care Unit, St Joseph Mercy Health System-Ann Arbor,
Ypsilanti, Michigan

CAROLYN D'AMBROSIO, MD, MS
Director, Harvard-Brigham and Women's Hospital; Pulmonary and Critical Care
Fellowship Program Faculty, Harvard Medical School, Boston, Massachusetts

MILES S. ELLENBY, MD, MS
Associate Professor, Departments of Pediatrics and Anesthesiology, Division of
Critical Care Medicine; Medical Director, Telemedicine Program, Doernbecher
Children's Hospital, Oregon Health & Science University, Portland, Oregon

JENNIFER A. FRONTERA, MD
Neurointensivist, Cerebrovascular Center, Neurologic Institute, Cleveland Clinic,
Cleveland, Ohio

ERKAN HASSAN, PharmD
Principal Scientist, Hospital to Home, Philips Healthcare, Baltimore, Maryland

THOMAS H. KALB, MD
Associate Medical Director, Advanced ICU Care Medical Group, New York, New York;
Associate Professor, Department of Medicine, North Shore/LIJ Hofstra School of
Medicine, Manhasset, New York

KATE E. KLEIN, ACNP
Nurse Practitioner, Cerebrovascular Center, Neurologic Institute, Cleveland Clinic,
Cleveland, Ohio

JAMES P. MARCIN, MD, MPH
Professor, Department of Pediatrics, Division of Critical Care, University of California
Davis Children's Hospital, Sacramento, California

JOSEPH S. MELTZER, MD
Associate Professor, Department of Anesthesiology and Perioperative Medicine,
Ronald Reagan UCLA Medical Center, David Geffen School of Medicine at UCLA,
Los Angeles, California

JAYANT K. RAIKHELKAR, MD
Fellow, Department of Cardiovascular Medicine, University Hospitals Case Medical
Center, Case Western Reserve University, Cleveland, Ohio

JAYASHREE RAIKHELKAR, MD
Assistant Professor of Anesthesiology, Department of Anesthesiology and Critical Care,
Emory University School of Medicine, Atlanta, Georgia

NAGARAJAN RAMAKRISHNAN, MD, MMM, FACP, FCCP, FCCM, FICCM
Director, Department of Critical Care Medicine, Apollo Hospitals, Chennai, India

PETER A. RASMUSSEN, MD
Cerebrovascular Center Director, Neurologic Institute, Cleveland Clinic, Cleveland, Ohio

H. NEAL REYNOLDS, MD
Associate Professor of Medicine, Division of Critical Care Medicine, R Adams Cowley
Shock Trauma Center, University of Maryland Medical Center, University of Maryland
School of Medicine, Baltimore, Maryland

HERB ROGOVE, DO, FCCM, FACP
C3O Telemedicine, Ojai, California

DANIEL M. ROLSTON, MD, MS
Clinical Instructor, Department of Emergency Medicine, Ronald Reagan UCLA Medical
Center, David Geffen School of Medicine at UCLA, Los Angeles, California

COREY SCURLOCK, MD, MBA
National Medical Director, Advanced ICU Care, New York, New York

KORY STETINA, CPC
Torch Health Solutions, San Diego, California

RAMESH VENKATARAMAN, MD, FACP, FCCP, FCCM
Senior Consultant and Academic Coordinator, Department of Critical Care Medicine,
Apollo Hospitals, Chennai, India

STACEY L. WINNERS, MSHS, RT(R)(CT), EMT-B
Mobile Stroke Treatment Unit Manager, Cerebrovascular Center, Neurologic Institute,
Cleveland Clinic, Cleveland, Ohio

Contents

> Critical care medicine is at a crossroads in which limited numbers of staff care for increasing numbers of patients as the population ages and use of ICUs increases. Also at this time health care spending must be curbed. The high-intensity intensivist staffing model has been linked to improved mortality, complications, and costs. Tele-ICU uses technology to implement this high-intensity staffing model in areas that are relatively underserved. When implemented correctly and in the right populations this technology has improved outcomes. Future studies regarding implementation, organization, staffing, and innovation are needed to determine the optimal use of this critical care professional enhanced technology.

> Telestroke and teleneurologic intensive care units (teleneuro-ICUs) optimize the diagnosis and treatment of neurologic emergencies. Establishment of a telestroke or teleneuro-ICU program relies on investment in experienced stroke and neurocritical care personnel as well as advanced telecommunications technologies. Telemanagement of neurologic emergencies can be standardized to improve outcomes, but it is essential to have a relationship with a tertiary care facility that can use endovascular, neurosurgical, and neurocritical care advanced therapies after stabilization. The next stage in telestroke/teleneuro-ICU management involves the use of mobile stroke units to shorten the time to treatment in neurocritically ill patients.

> Telemedicine has been increasingly used in the intensive care unit setting (Tele-ICU) for providing care. Given the shortage of qualified intensivists and critical care nurses in the United States and the ever-increasing demand for intensive care services, Tele-ICU has been proposed as a strategy to bridge this supply/demand gap. The Tele-ICU staffing model provides for many important outcome benefits that have been evaluated over the years by several studies. In this review, the authors summarize the existing evidence and identify areas where further evaluation is warranted.

Disasters and emergencies lead to an overburdened health care system after the event, so additional telemedicine support can improve patient outcomes. If telemedicine is going to become an integral part of disaster response, there needs to be improved preparation for the use of telemedicine technologies. Telemedicine can improve patient triage, monitoring, access to specialists, health care provider burnout, and disaster recovery. However, the evidence for telemedicine and tele-intensive care in the disaster setting is limited, and it should be further studied to identify situations in which it is the most clinically effective and cost-effective.

This article explores the hypothesis that a telemedicine intensive care unit (Tele-ICU) platform is uniquely suited to facilitate quality performance improvement (PI). This article addresses some substantial hurdles to overcome that may limit the effectiveness of a Tele-ICU platform to achieve PI objectives. Lastly, this article describes the author's experience with a PI project to improve ventilator management conducted via a Tele-ICU hub interacting with 11 geographically dispersed ICUs. Using this example to illustrate the concepts, the author hopes to shed some light on the successes and lessons learned so as to generate best-practice guidelines for Tele-ICU-directed PI initiatives.

Telemedicine technologies involve real-time, live, interactive video and audio communication and allow pediatric critical care physicians to have a virtual presence at the bedsides of critically ill children. Telemedicine use is increasing in remote emergency departments, inpatient wards, and intensive care units for pediatric care. Hospitals and physicians that use telemedicine technologies provide higher quality of care, are more efficient in resource use with improved cost-effectiveness, and have high satisfaction among patients, parents, and remote providers. More research will result in improved access to pediatric critical care expertise.

Severe sepsis remains a significant medical problem affecting up to 18 million individuals worldwide. Mortality remains high ranging between 28% and 50%. Owing to this and the time-sensitive nature of this disease state, early identification and prompt interventions are necessary to improve outcomes. Technology associated with telemedicine may help in screening, identifying, and monitoring the attainment of the severe sepsis bundle elements in a timely manner. However, the heterogeneity of systemic inflammatory response syndrome and clinical assessment necessary to diagnose and assess patients with severe sepsis makes technology alone insufficient to improve the outcomes in these patients.

The Impact of Telemedicine in Cardiac Critical Care   305

Jayashree Raikhelkar and Jayant K. Raikhelkar

Telemedicine was recognized in the 1970s as a legitimate entity for applying the use of modern information and communications technologies to the delivery of health services. Telecardiology is one of the fastest growing fields in telemedicine. The advancement of technologies and Web-based applications has allowed better transmission of health care delivery. This article discusses current advancements, the scope of tele-medicine in cardiology, and its application to the critically ill. The impact of telecardiology consultation continues to evolve and includes many promising applications with potential positive implications for admission rates, morbidity, and mortality.

Practice Challenges of Intensive Care Unit Telemedicine   319

Herb Rogove and Kory Stetina

For more than 20 years, a 100-year-old state-based system for medical licensure has not progressed commensurate with the level of 21st century technology development. Despite government and nongovernment organizational attempts, each state maintains a process of variable and time-consuming requirements with lack of reciprocity. Lack of available reimbursement for Tele-ICU physician services is thought to be a long-standing and significant barrier to the rapid adoption of Tele-ICU programs. By reviewing the reimbursement guidelines for telehealth ser-vices across all major patient financial classes, a model is discussed for developing financial projections to determine exactly what reimbursement is available for Tele-ICU programs.

Options for Tele-Intensive Care Unit Design: Centralized Versus Decentralized and Other Considerations: It Is Not Just a "Another Black Sedan"   335

H. Neal Reynolds and Joseph J. Bander

This article seeks to assist physicians or administrators considering estab-lishing a Tele-ICU. Owing to an apparent domination of the Tele-ICU field by a single vendor, some may believe that there is only one design option. In fact, there are many alternative design formats that do not require the consumer to possess high-level technical expertise. As when purchasing any major item, if the consumer can formulate basic concepts of design and research the various vendors, then the consumer can develop the Tele-ICU system best for their facility, finances, availability of staff, coverage model, and quality metric goals.

CRITICAL CARE CLINICS

ISSUE OF RELATED INTEREST

Critical Care Nursing Clinics of North America, December 2014 (Vol. 26, No. 4)
Quality
Barbara Leeper and Rosemary Luquire, *Editors*
Available at: http://www.ccnursing.theclinics.com/

NOW AVAILABLE FOR YOUR iPhone and iPad

Preface

Telemedicine in the ICU

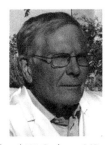 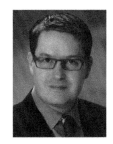

Richard W. Carlson, MD, PhD   Corey Scurlock, MD, MBA
Editors

Critical care medicine, like no other field in medicine, is in a period of limited resources. This comes at a time when the demand for critical care expertise is starting a period of exponential growth, as baby-boomers age and increasingly need the ICU. All of this is occurring when health care resources are scarce and the US debt to gross domestic product ratio is at an all time high. This has led many to attempt to find novel ways to meet these shortages and to contain costs. Telemedicine in the ICU, or Tele-ICU, is one of these methods that may not only help solve staffing issues but also lead to new and different ways of care that more heavily rely on artificial intelligence, alerting systems, and computerized algorithms to help intervene on patients in a more timely fashion, perhaps even before they become unstable. These alerting and reminding systems may have added benefit in increasing compliance with best practices and reducing medical error. Given that critical care medicine itself is a relatively new field in medicine, telemedicine to provide critical care is even more recent and can truly be considered a field in infancy. This movement has led to tele-ICUs increasingly being studied in literature, with different models and methods offering different results. In this issue of *Critical Care Clinics*, there is a focus on telemedicine in the ICU in a broad sense with recent literature around it along with more detailed specialty-based overviews of specific implications for it from sepsis to pediatrics. This issue also has perspectives in relation to obstacles in organizational structure and governmental issues that also affect the field.

We are fortunate to have the expertise of a wide variety of authorities in this area, who have dedicated their time and knowledge in helping us construct this issue. It is always an honor and a joy to work with such high-quality experts and to learn from not only their submissions to this issue but also their unique perspective and experience in the field. We wish to offer our deepest thanks not only to them but also to

Crit Care Clin 31 (2015) ix–x
http://dx.doi.org/10.1016/j.ccc.2015.01.001
0749-0704/15/$ – see front matter © 2015 Published by Elsevier Inc.

criticalcare.theclinics.com

our editorial staff, including Patrick Manley at Elsevier, who helped us to ensure deadlines and to produce a high-quality product.

Richard W. Carlson, MD, PhD
Medical Intensive Care Unit
Maricopa Medical Center
Phoenix, AZ 85008, USA

College of Medicine
Mayo Clinic
Scottsdale, AZ, USA

University of Arizona College of Medicine
Phoenix, AZ, USA

Corey Scurlock, MD, MBA
Advanced ICU Care
747 Third Avenue, Suite 28 A
New York, NY 10017, USA

E-mail addresses:
RichardW_Carlson@dmgaz.org (R.W. Carlson)
cscurlock@icumedicine.com (C. Scurlock)

Telemedicine in the Intensive Care Unit

State of the Art

Corey Scurlock, MD, MBA[a],*, Carolyn D'Ambrosio, MD, MS[b]

KEYWORDS

- Tele-ICU • Intensivist staffing • Quality improvement • Technology in medicine
- Health care finances • Checklists

KEY POINTS

- Critical care medicine is at an important moment in its history.
- Leveraging technology and relative intensivist populations through telemedicine is a way of helping with this crisis and allowing patients in hospitals without intensivists on site to have state-of-the-art care.
- Telemedicine in the ICU, although an infant field, does just that, taking advantage of intensivist population imbalances while also leveraging technology to help meet the demands of the critically ill across the nation.

The Future is Today
        —*Sir William Osler*

THE CHALLENGE AHEAD

Critical care medicine like all of medicine is at an important crossroads; however, it faces unique challenges like no other medical specialty. Two of the biggest challenges critical care medicine faces are a high debt to gross domestic product ratio that will force the US health care system to contain costs, and an aging population that will increasingly need intensive care unit (ICU) resources. This comes at a time in which there are limited numbers of intensivists, and for that matter limited total critical care professionals.

Health care in the United States is the most expensive in the world and the cost of critical care services is not an insignificant fraction of this sum. In 2005, the cost of

Disclosure Statement: The authors have no financial disclosures.
[a] Advanced ICU Care, 747 Third Avenue, Suite 28 A, New York, NY 10017, USA;
[b] Harvard-Brigham and Women's Hospital, Pulmonary and Critical Care Fellowship Program Faculty, Harvard Medical School, Boston, MA 02115, USA
* Corresponding author.
E-mail address: cscurlock@icumedicine.com

Crit Care Clin 31 (2015) 187–195
http://dx.doi.org/10.1016/j.ccc.2014.12.001
0749-0704/15/$ – see front matter © 2015 Elsevier Inc. All rights reserved.

providing critical care in the United States was estimated at 81.7 billion annually, accounting for 0.66% of gross domestic product, greater than 10% of hospital costs, and 4% of national health expenditures.[1] This is a time in which the population is aging, placing an increasing strain on current resources. The percentage of the population in the United States older than 65 will increase 50% by 2020 and will double by 2030.[2] Importantly, as the population ages the need for ICU resources becomes increasingly common with patients older than 64 years of age using the ICU at 3.5 times the rate of the population younger than 64 years of age. Clearly, the demand for ICU staff and expertise will continue to increase in the coming years.

Compounding the high demand is that there is a profound lack of ICU staff, particularly intensivists, on the horizon. For a variety of reasons internal medicine residents have little interest in critical care.[3,4] For critical care physicians with surgical or anesthesia training, most will practice critical care part-time or in only a limited basis. In addition, many critical care trained physicians of all backgrounds either seek not to practice critical care full-time or retire early from the field secondary to burnout-related issues.[5] In the original COMPACCS study it was revealed that only one-third of Americans in the ICU were treated by a critical care physician, with many of those physicians practicing only part-time.[6,7] Never was this shortage more strongly felt than in the implementation and eventual failure or the original Leapfrog recommendations. Based on a few observational trials, the Leapfrog group concluded that the care of ICU patients would greatly improve if intensivists provided their care.[7] Unfortunately, this recommendation could not be implemented broadly secondary to manpower shortages.[8] From this we learned definitively that with current conditions, intensivists cannot take care of every patient in every ICU in the country. In 2002, the Institute of Medicine reported on health inequities in the United States with access to care being a significant contributor.[9] Several conditions in critically ill patients have better outcomes if appropriate care is given early on, such as sepsis, acute respiratory distress syndrome, venous thromboembolism, and acute coronary syndrome. Having access to a hospital does not necessarily mean having access to state-of-the-art care. For critically ill patients variations in the quality of health care can have devastating consequences, such as worse outcomes and longer hospital and ICU stays.[10] In 2011, the first baby-boomers began to retire, setting the stage for the moment at which the population begins to diverge and the health care system will have to make choices and important questions have to be asked and answered:

- How will we meet the staffing demands placed on our system by an aging population with increasingly limited financial resources?
- How can we use technology to continue to advance our field?
- Can we use technology to help us find new ways to improve process, enforce best practices, and identify acutely ill patients more readily?
- How do we improve our ability to reduce medical error and cost?

Multiple ideas have been pushed forward on how to solve these shortages. Such solutions as training hospitalists in critical care, adding more advanced practice practitioners (APPs) to the critical care workforce, and increasing the number of trained critical care physicians have all been suggested. Given that the problem is so large, an amalgamation of these ideas will ultimately be the solution. Another idea that has been suggested is that the role of the intensivist may evolve into leading teams of health care professionals, whether that be working with APP teams, or helping hospitalists in the care of critically ill patients in a consultative role. What is clear is that quality, safety, monetary, and efficiency demands may force these changes on intensivists rather than any internal forces within our specialty.

We live in an increasingly urbanized and technological world with rapid and newer forms of communication evolving and constantly changing our society. Perhaps telemedicine or tele-ICU may solve this supply/demand imbalance. The rest of this article focuses on the use of telemedicine in the ICU. Sections on its creation and evolution, data in terms of the medical literature, and then keys to success in its implementation and correct usage are discussed.

THE EVOLUTION OF TELEMEDICINE

The most basic definition of ICU telemedicine or tele-ICU involves using technology to provide critical care services from remote areas, and stems from the Latin word "medicus" and the Greek "tele," literally meaning "to heal at a distance." Telemedicine was first developed in the 1970s and described at that time as "applying the use of modern information and communications technologies for the delivery of health services."[11] In the early 1980s tele-ICU was first described by Grundy and colleagues.[12] This has evolved into two-way audio-video technology that links remote critical practitioners (nurses, APPs, and physicians) to remote areas with continuous monitoring and sharing of information.

Modern telemedicine in the ICU typically occurs in monitoring centers that house intensivists, critical care trained APPs, and critical care nurses. This represents the closed model of tele-ICUs, which at this time is by far the most common type of tele-ICU. At these monitoring centers, patients at remote hospitals are monitored either in a continuous 24/7 fashion or during nighttime hours and weekends when there is a dearth of staff. In general, these monitoring centers tend to be clustered in urban areas with high population densities of intensivists. This allows for leveraging of technology and population dynamics to provide critical care resources to areas that are relatively underserved. Given that nighttime work has been highly correlated with burnout, it seems that using technology to help reduce this burden would be of immense help in sustaining our critical workforce.[13]

Tele-ICU also has the potential to provide better outcomes by the use of alerting systems to detect early physiologic deterioration (ie, sepsis, stroke, myocardial infarction), alerting and reminding systems to address best practices, and increasing patient access to dedicated intensivists. Thus far the literature has been mixed in regards to outcomes with multiple studies showing enhanced outcomes, whereas others yield little to no benefit. One must also be mindful that there are significant cultural, financial, and organizational barriers to implementation of telemedicine broadly.

Modern tele-ICU (ie, closed model monitoring centers) began in earnest in 2000 but really had more regular adoption starting in 2003. The years of 2003 to 2013 were a period of rapid growth for tele-ICUs. According to Kahn and colleagues,[14] the number of tele-ICUs increased from 16 (0.4% of all hospitals) in 2003 to 213 (4.6% of all hospitals) (P<.001). This represented a staggering mean annual increase of 61% per year.[14] In parallel, the number of ICU beds being covered by a tele-ICU swelled from 598 in 2003, to 5,799 in 2010. Surprisingly, this occurred throughout the country with no single region of the country having predominance. When looking at the characteristics of these hospitals, most (50.7%) were in the mid-size range (100–400 total beds) and most (91%) were nonprofit. This trend seemed to strengthen in the second 5 years of the study with 63.5% of the hospitals being in the mid-size range of 100 to 400 total beds. Anyone familiar with basic marketing will have heard of the Rogers' Model of Diffusion of Innovation (**Fig. 1**) in which once a new technology or product is created it goes through several notable phases (see **Fig. 1**). Medicine has rules and laws that apply to it, like any other industry. Tele-ICU is obviously on some portion

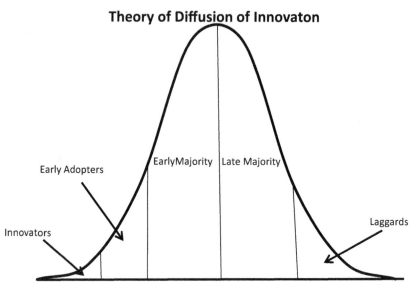

Fig. 1. Rogers' model of diffusion of innovation. (*Adapted from* Rogers EM. Diffusion of innovations. 5th edition. New York: Free Press; 2003.)

of this curve and that exact point remains debatable. Given its size, breadth, and longevity, tele-ICU has clearly passed the phase of early adoption. To truly be successful any technology must pass the second phase of early adopters to reach the early majority. This is critical in reaching large segments of the population. Whether or not tele-ICU is at the early majority phase is still up for debate but given the increasing role technology plays in our lives and workspace that jump seems extraordinarily likely.

DATA

Access to intensivists and high-intensity staffing models are associated with reductions in ICU and in-hospital mortality.[15] This was seen most recently in a meta-analysis of 52 composite studies analyzing high-intensity staffing models versus low-intensity staffing models. In 34 of these studies, mortality was lower in the high-intensity staffing cohort (risk ratio = 0.83; 95% confidence interval [CI], 0.70–0.99). A second meta-analysis in this area found similar results with high-intensity staffing models associated with a reduction in hospital mortality (risk ratio = 0.71; 95% CI, 0.62–0.82).[16] In both of these studies, a major limitation is that there has been little to no analysis of community hospitals, with a preponderance of the centers being studied consisting of academic medical centers. A further limitation is that, almost by definition these are observational studies. Although observational studies have been helpful in the literature (ie, the causal relationship between smoking and cancer in the 1960s), they can be prone to bias and error. In addition, given that these studies are meta-analyses they are subject to publication bias. The addition of nighttime intensivists has had mixed results in the literature, potentially helping in units with low-intensity staffing models without the same effect seen in high-intensity staffing models.[17,18] All of this leaves one to ponder what effect the addition of tele-ICU has to high-intensity staffing models, low-intensity staffing models, and also its effect in academic medical centers and the community.

Three recent studies have addressed this issue in the academic setting. The first consists of a before-after study published in 2011.[19] This study was conducted at a single academic medical center from 2005 to 2007 across a variety of types of ICUs including three medical, three surgical, and one mixed cardiovascular. It analyzed more than 6000 patients and was specifically powered to detect a 3.5% improvement in mortality with a significance level of 0.05. Of note, at the time of the study a daily goal sheet was also introduced at the bedside. This clearly has important patient safety implications.[20] Importantly, this study looked at care processes around the implementation of a tele-ICU, and it was novel in that approach. After the implementation of the tele-ICU, hospital mortality dropped from 13.6% to 11.8% with an odds ratio of 0.4 (95% CI, 0.31–0.52; $P = .005$). A similar trend was seen for ICU mortality, which dropped from 10.7% to 8.6%, with odds ratio of 0.37 (95% CI, 0.28–0.49; $P = .003$). Also, at the same time, ICU length-of-stay (LOS) decreased to 4.5 days compared with 6.4 days preimplementation ($P<.001$). This meant that quality improved (ie, reductions in mortality) while cost presumably also decreased (ie, reduced LOS). To understand these differences, the authors analyzed compliance with best practices. They found that the addition of the tele-ICU was associated with higher compliance with deep venous thrombosis and stress ulcer prophylaxis. This was coupled with a dramatic reduction in ventilator-associated pneumonia and catheter-related bloodstream infections.

Analysis was also performed by time of admission to look for diurnal cycles in care. It was presumed that the tele-ICU would only have impact at night because this academic center had intensivists with teams of residents and fellows rounding during the day with residents on call at the bedside at night. The tele-ICU as an isolated intervention was associated with shorter hospital LOS (hazard ratio, 1.61; 95% CI, 1.35–1.92; $P<.001$) and similar results were seen with ICU LOS and days on mechanical ventilation for patients admitted after 8:00 PM. Finally, in terms of responding to alerts and alarms for physiologic instability, the tele-ICU team prompted the bedside team on average of 1.7 times per patient per day. Obviously this study has important limitations in that it was at a single academic medical center and was also unblinded. There was also a higher level of acuity in the patients after the implementation of the tele-ICU possibly reflecting higher rates of transfer of high-acuity patients into a quaternary care center.

In 2014, these same authors analyzed 118,990 patients admitted to ICUs between 2003 and 2008, across 56 ICUs in 32 hospitals from 19 US health care systems in a pre/post assessment of implementing an ICU telemedicine program.[21] This study was notable for not only its size and statistical power but also for its scope, given that it was the first study to look at the effect of telemedicine across the United States. After the implementation of a tele-ICU, ICU LOS shortened by a factor of 20% (95% CI, 19%–22%; $P<.001$) and hospital LOS was reduced by a factor of 15% for patients coming through the ICU (95% CI, 14%–17%; $P<.001$). In this study there were six processes that were associated with improved outcomes (**Box 1**). Not surprisingly many of these items revolve around early involvement by an intensivist, computer alerting and reminding systems, and the use of data to drive quality improvement in a collaborative manner.

The most recent study to look at quality was an observational pre/post study published in 2014 on the effects of implementing a tele-ICU across eight ICUs in the US Department of Veterans Affairs health care system from 2011 to 2012.[22] The ICUs monitored were a combination of medical, surgical, and mixed medical-surgical. When matching these tele-ICUs to control ICUs there was no statistically significant difference in ICU, in-hospital, or 30-day mortality. Furthermore, there was no

---

Box 1
Factors associated with improved outcomes after implementing Tele-ICUs

A. Intensivists performing review of the care plan within 1 hour of admission

B. Frequent and collaborative review and use of performance data

C. Implementation-related increases in the rates of adherence to best practices

D. Shorter response times for laboratory alerts and alarms for physiologic instability

E. Performance of interdisciplinary rounds

F. Effectiveness of the institution's ICU committee

---

difference in LOS compared with control ICUs. When looked at in isolation, one might conclude that there are no added benefits to tele-ICUs; however, the mortality rate in control and intervention groups was very low and it may have been difficult to detect a difference. In addition the acuity of the patients was not very high compared with other tele-ICU studies with low severity of illness and not many of the patients were mechanically ventilated. Finally, the Veterans Affairs health system has a heavy amount of intensivist staffing, infrastructure, and support that may not lend itself to the most benefit from a tele-ICU monitoring system in the background, thus making it difficult to show improvement in even the best designed studies.

KEYS TO SUCCESS
Understanding Local Culture

In the world of tele-ICU, one could not find a truer statement than the mantra "All politics are local." Understanding local culture, care, and referral patterns is paramount when implementing and maintaining a tele-ICU. Human relationships play a very important role in making this technology work at its highest level. In a nursing survey study of 72 nurses with an average of 5 years ICU experience, 79% believed that knowing the tele-ICU physician is important.[23] This undoubtedly played a role in that only 44% of those same ICU nurses regularly incorporated the tele-ICU recommendations. This occurred despite 72% of them admitting that they believed the tele-ICU improved survival. When looking at these data, there is somewhat of a disconnect in this study and although not stated implicitly in the study, lack of personal relations had to play a role. Other than looking at medical residence acceptance of telemedicine, these studies have not been replicated in physicians.[24] However, clearly physician acceptance of this same technology-enabled service and human relations with this cohort are also vitally important. Just as with any other medium, without good collaboration and cooperation on both sides of the technology, care cannot be optimized.

Driving Process Improvement

Given the rich operational environment of ICUs combined with the tremendous data that automated processes bring, the tele-ICU offers much in the way of driving process improvement. A recent example of this was published in the literature in 2014 by Kalb and colleagues.[25] This study was unique in that it looked at a single process in relation to quality improvement that a tele-ICU implemented across several hospitals in disparate locations. In this process the tele-ICU intensivist directed "ventilator rounds" during off-hour times with the local on-site respiratory therapists. Before implementation of these ventilator rounds there was poor adherence to low tidal volume therapy (mean 29.5% ± 18.2% with range of 10%–69%). After 9 months or approximately three quarters there was statistically significant improvement in this data point (mean, 44.9 ± 15.7%), which was maintained even after the study finished. Importantly, reductions in the Acute Physiology and Chronic Health Evaluation IV ventilator duration (0.92 ± 0.28; −15.8%; $P<.05$) and mortality ratios (0.94 vs 0.67; $P<.04$) also achieved statistical significance by the third quarter postimplementation of this quality improvement project.

Developing Research

Like any other field, high-impact research is needed to ensure the value of a tele-ICU. Importantly this was recognized, and in a 2-day summit in March 2010, a working group of clinicians and researchers reviewed the current literature in regards to tele-ICU and setting a research agenda for future studies involving telemedicine in the ICU.[26] Notably, this group asked that in future research a novel standardized framework be used that involved having preimplementation data and having a more narrow and predefined term for telemedicine in the ICU. The key knowledge gaps as defined by this group involved structure, process, and outcome (**Box 2**).

SUMMARY

Critical care medicine is at an important moment in its history. Divergent forces of population growth, cost containment, and limited supply of intensivists have forced the issue of looking at alternative means of helping to meet the demands required of the critical care workforce. Leveraging technology and relative intensivist populations through telemedicine is a way of helping with this crisis and allowing patients in hospitals without intensivists onsite to have state-of-the-art care. Telemedicine in the ICU,

---

Box 2
Key knowledge gaps and areas of focus for future research

Research items related to structure

- Organization of the telemedicine
- Organization of ICUs being monitored
- Optimal staffing
- Optimal work environments
- Readiness to change

Research items related to process

- Optimal delivery of telemedicine
- Evidenced-based care
- Education regarding telemedicine
- Areas of innovation in telemedicine

Research items related to outcomes

- Mortality
- Morbidity
- Cost outcomes
- Operator satisfaction
- Patient satisfaction

---

although an infant field, does just that, taking advantage of intensivist population imbalances while also leveraging technology to help meet the demands of the critically ill across the nation. This novel way of taking care of patients may also have new and important implications in helping to reduce morbidity, mortality, and potentially reduce cost. Much of this will revolve around data and looking at processes within ICUs and the proper environment to implement this technology. Further studies and a unified research agenda are needed to help solidify and find its ultimate correct setting in the field.

REFERENCES

1. NHE Fact Sheet. Available at: https://www.cms.gove/NationalHealthExpendData/25_NHE_Fact_Sheet.asp#TOPOFPAGE. Accessed August 2, 2014.
2. Available at: http://www.census.gov/prod/2010pubs/p25-1138.pdf. Accessed August 3, 2014.
3. Lorin S, Heffner J, Carson S. Attitudes and perceptions of internal medicine residents regarding pulmonary and critical care subspecialty training. Chest 2005; 127:630–6.
4. Kovitz KL. Pulmonary and critical care: the unattractive specialty. Chest 2005; 127:1085–7.
5. US Department of Health and Human Services, Health Resources and Services Administration. Report to Congress: the critical care workforce; a study of the supply and demand for critical care physicians. Washington, DC: Requested by Congress 2003, released May 10, 2006.
6. Angus DC, Kelley MA, Schmitz RJ, et al. Caring for the critically ill patient: current and projected workforce requirements for care of the critically ill and patients with pulmonary disease. Can we meet the requirements of an aging population? JAMA 2000;284:2762–70.
7. Pronovost PJ, Thompson DA, Holzmueller CG, et al. The organization of intensive care unit physician services. Crit Care Med 2007;35:2256–61.
8. Angus DC, Shorr AF, White A, et al. Critical care delivery in the United States: distribution of services and compliance with Leapfrog recommendations. Crit Care Med 2006;34:1016–24.
9. Smedley BD, Stith AY, Nelson AR. Unequal treatment: confronting racial and ethnic disparities in healthcare. Washington, DC: National Academies Press; 2002.
10. Martin GS. Healthcare disparities in critically ill patients. In: Vincent J-L, editor. Yearbook of intensive care and emergency medicine, vol. 2006. New York: Springer; 2006. p. 778–85.
11. Strehle EM, Shabde N. One hundred years of telemedicine: does this technology have a place in paediatrics? Arch Dis Child 2006;91(12):956–9.
12. Grundy BL, Jones PK, Lovitt A. Telemedicine in critical care: problems in design, implementation, and assessment. Crit Care Med 1982;10(7):471–5.
13. Embriaco N, Azoulay E, Barrau K, et al. High level of burnout in intensivists: prevalence and associated factors. Am J Respir Crit Care Med 2007;175:686–92.
14. Kahn JM, Cicero BD, Wallace DJ, et al. Adoption of ICU telemedicine in the United States. Crit Care Med 2014;42:362–8.
15. Wilcox MR, Chong CA, Niven DJ, et al. Do intensivist staffing patterns influence hospital mortality following ICU admission? A systematic review and meta-analysis. Crit Care Med 2013;4(10):2253–74.
16. Gajic O, Afessa B, Hanson AC, et al. Effect of 24-hour mandatory versus on-demand critical care specialist presence on quality of care and family and

provider satisfaction in the intensive care unit of a teaching hospital. Crit Care Med 2008;36:36–44.

17. Walalce DJ, Angus DC, Barnato AE, et al. Nightime intensivist staffing and mortality among critically ill patients. N Engl J Med 2012;366(22):2093–101.

18. Raikhelkar J, Scurlock C, Kopec I. Nightime intensivist staffing. N Engl J Med 2012;367(10):971.

19. Lilly CM, Cody S, Zhao H, et al. Hospital mortality, length of stay, and preventable complications among critically ill patients before and after tele-ICU reengineering of critical care processes. JAMA 2011;305(21):2175–83.

20. Pronovost P, Needham D, Berenholtz S, et al. An intervention to decrease catheter-related bloodstream infections in the ICU. N Engl J Med 2006;26: 2725–32.

21. Lilly CM, McLaughlin JM, Zhao H, et al. A multicenter study of ICU telemedicine reengineering of adult critical care. Chest 2014;145(3):500–7.

22. Nassar BS, Vaughan-Sarrazin MS, Jian L, et al. Impact of an intensive care unit telemedicine program on patient outcomes in an integrated health care system. JAMA Intern Med 2014;174(7):1160–7.

23. Mullen-Forting M, DiMartino J, Entrikin L, et al. Bedside nurses' perceptions of intensive care unit telemedicine. Am J Crit Care 2012;21:24–31.

24. Coletti C, Elliot DJ, Zubrow MT. Resident perceptions of a tele-intensive care unit implementation. Telemed J E Health 2010;16:894–7.

25. Kalb T, Raikhelkar J, Meyer S, et al. A multicenter population-based effectiveness study of teleintensive care unit-directed ventilator rounds demonstrating improved adherence to a protective lung strategy, decreased ventilator duration, and decreased intensive care unit mortality. J Crit Care 2014;29(4):e7–14.

26. Kahn JM, Hill NS, Lilly CM, et al. The research agenda in ICU telemedicine: a statement from the Critical Care Societies Collaborative. Chest 2011;140:230–8.

Teleneurocritical Care and Telestroke

Kate E. Klein, ACNP, Peter A. Rasmussen, MD, Stacey L. Winners, MSHS, RT(R)(CT), EMT-B, Jennifer A. Frontera, MD*

KEYWORDS

- Telestroke • Tele-ICU • Teleneuro-ICU • tPA • Mobile stroke unit

KEY POINTS

- Telestroke and teleneurologic intensive care units (teleneuro-ICUs) are now part of mainstream clinical practice and are safe, reliable, cost-saving strategies that improve the timely response to neurologic ICU emergencies, decrease hospital lengths of stay, and improve functional outcomes.
- Telestroke and teleneuro-ICUs reduce disparities in access to expert care, ensuring that no hospital remains underserved and no patients with acute stroke receive suboptimal care.
- The ideal telestroke/teleneuro-ICU system is one that includes a high-quality, real-time, encrypted, audiovideo teleconferencing system; neuroimaging integration; mobility for site independence; decision and technical support features; electronic medical record integration; and billing and documentation that can be implemented across the World Wide Web.
- Mobile stroke treatment units are revolutionizing stroke care by providing prehospital timely, accurate stroke care, thus providing patients with the best possible recovery outcomes from their strokes.

INTRODUCTION

Neurologic injury of any type occurring in the young and elderly requires timely evaluation, diagnosis, and treatment in both the acute and postacute phases of recovery to optimize functional outcome. As the proportion of older people and life expectancy increase throughout the world,[1,2] the incidence of stroke and neurocritical care emergencies is expected to increase concomitantly. Effective treatments should not be withheld because of age unless there is compelling evidence to suggest that risk is

Disclosures: The authors have nothing to disclose.
Cerebrovascular Center, Neurological Institute, Cleveland Clinic, 9500 Euclid Avenue, Cleveland, OH 44195, USA
* Corresponding author. Cerebrovascular Center, Cleveland Clinic Foundation, 9500 Euclid Avenue, S80, Cleveland, OH 44195.
E-mail address: frontej@ccf.org

greater than benefit. Approximately 30% of acute strokes, for example, occur in those more than 80 years of age.[1,2] In an adjusted controlled comparison of outcomes trials, better outcomes with thrombolytic therapy, intravenous (IV) tissue plasminogen activator (tPA), did not depend on age.[3] Knowledge of acute stroke and neurocritical care is evolving rapidly with specialized stroke and neurocritical care expertise advancing accurate assessment and delivery of therapies.[4] Worldwide, stroke (including ischemic stroke, subarachnoid hemorrhage [SAH], and intracerebral hemorrhage) is a major public health problem. An estimated 15.3 million strokes occur worldwide.[5] In the United States a stroke occurs every 40 seconds, and every 4 minutes someone dies from a stroke.[6] In the United States stroke is the fourth leading cause of death and the number 1 cause of disability. Among survivors, 15% to 30% are permanently disabled and 20% require institutional care, incurring an estimated cost of $65 billion annually.[7–9]

During the acute phase, a neurocritically ill patient's recovery to independence is contingent on the timing of treatment delivery. The saying that time is brain has taken on new meaning with the advent of clinically effective treatments, such as IV thrombolysis with recombinant tPA (IV tPA) for acute ischemic stroke,[10] mechanical embolectomy for large-vessel ischemic stroke, coagulopathy reversal for intracranial hemorrhage (ICH), immediate and aggressive treatment of seizures, prompt aneurysm repair for patients with SAH, intracranial pressure (ICP) management for patients with traumatic brain injury, and timely surgical decompression for malignant cerebral edema and intracerebral hemorrhage.[11] In patients with ischemic stroke, for every hour without blood flow, 120 million neurons are lost, and every minute, 1.9 million neurons are lost.[12] For each stroke, it is estimated that 1.2 billion neurons die, which accelerates aging by 36 years.[12] Immediate intervention with IV tPA can spare penumbral infarction and limit the neurologic damage of stroke, if delivered promptly. In patients with SAH, the greatest risk of aneurysm rebleed occurs within the first 24 hours of rupture. Rebleed significantly increases the risk of death or severe disability, but can be treated by prompt aneurysm repair and attenuated by administration of antifibrinolytics such as aminocaproic acid and tranexamic acid.[13,14] Similarly, in the case of seizures, if treatment is delivered within 30 minutes, 80% of seizures are aborted with a first-line agent. In contrast, if treatment is delayed for 2 hours, the response to antiepileptics decreases by more than half to less than 40%.[15] The more time that goes by without treatment, the more likely the patient is to continue seizing, develop status epilepticus, and require intubation, and therefore to develop all the potential problems associated with respiratory failure.[16] Arguably, these neurologic emergencies are more time sensitive than even acute myocardial infarction, which has traditionally been the focus of time-sensitive management. Even though these evidence-based treatments have been available for more than a decade, most neurocritically ill patients do not receive these highly time-sensitive treatments.[17] In most countries there is a shortage of specialists in neurosciences, and available neurologists and neurosurgeons are clustered in metropolitan, urban areas.[18] IV tPA, in particular, is given to only 2% to 7% of eligible patients.[19] The optimal model of care for responding to acute neurologic injury and potential malignant sequelae is one that offers timely physical and imaging assessment, evaluation with treatment recommendations by an expert clinical neuroscientist, followed by stabilization and close observation and follow-up treatment in a neurologic intensive care unit (neuro-ICU). Having this model of care available to all neurocritically ill patients is a challenge given the cost of technology, shortage of available intensivists, and lack of overnight coverage that would best provide safe, high-quality initial and ongoing care to patients.

BENEFITS OF TELESTROKE/TELENEUROLOGIC INTENSIVE CARE UNITS

Telemedicine, first introduced in the 1950s,[20] is a subset of a broader scope of distance health care delivery technologies. It can provide continuous intensive care unit (ICU) monitoring and consultation from an intensivist at a remote location. To date, continuous ICU monitoring has shown variable impacts on outcomes, from no benefit to modest improvement in ICU mortality, length of stay (LOS), and preventable complications.[21] Telemedicine applied in a different paradigm, coined telestroke in 1999,[22] uses bidirectional communication to allow stroke specialists to offer time-sensitive evaluation of patients presenting with stroke symptoms. Telestroke technology can be applied in prehospital and emergency department (ED) settings, as well as in the ICU setting for monitoring and responding to postacute emergencies. The overarching goal of telestroke and teleneuro-ICU is to provide all patients with neurologic injury with the best possible outcome with access to the right provider, the right therapy, at the right time, and the right facility for their care and recovery. Other benefits of telestroke and teleneuro-ICU are listed in **Box 1**. The initial main impetus for the application of telestroke to stroke care was to overcome disparities of stroke care delivery and barriers preventing timely determination of stroke symptom cause and delivery of IV tPA within protocol guidelines.[23] In addition to the low delivery rates of tPA, other treatments for ischemic stroke, including early antiplatelet therapy, intra-arterial (IA) tPA, endovascular mechanical thrombectomy, and surgical decompression for malignant edema, continue to be inaccessible to most stroke victims.[24] Barriers to these treatments include poor community awareness of stroke symptoms, narrow time window of effective intervention with tPA, lack of specialized stroke services in

---

Box 1
Benefits of telestroke and teleneuro-ICU

Benefits

Improves EMS access to victims of neurologic injury

Optimizes use of IV tPA in ischemic stroke

- Accurate identification of candidates for tPA

- Improves clinician comfort with tPA

- Decreases symptom onset to treatment time

- Delivery of tPA without protocol violation

- Increases rate of tPA delivery

Increases access to expert neurologic consultation

Identifies candidates for endovascular stroke therapies

Improves access to specialists and emergency management in the care of neurologic injuries

Improves patient outcomes

Faster transfers for emergent cases

Improves patient and caregiver satisfaction

Mitigates malpractice risk

Increases potential for participation in clinical trials

Facilitates accurate disposition

Abbreviation: EMS, emergency medical system.

underserved areas, shortage of specialty stroke-trained physicians and caregivers, lack of obligate neurologic specialty coverage in EDs, concern for intracerebral hemorrhage risk using tPA, long distance to a primary or comprehensive stroke centers, limited neurosurgical access, and insufficient reimbursement for acute stroke consultations via telestroke.[24–27] The severe effects of stroke and overcoming these barriers have led to the development of the stroke unit concept and application of telestroke systems into the mainstream of stroke care.[28] Telestroke's greatest impact has been in decreasing regional stroke care disparities by allowing rural settings access to expertise from specialty centers.[29] Nonspecialized regional hospitals and their patients stand to benefit considerably by collaborating with comprehensive or primary stroke center neurologists using telestroke. A recent cost-effectiveness study found that comparing no telestroke network to a network with a single hub and 7 spoke facilities resulted in 45 more people treated with tPA, 20 more patients treated with endovascular stroke therapies, and 5 more patients recovering to independence and discharged home per 1000 patients with acute ischemic stroke per year.[30]

Beyond acute treatments of stroke, patients with other neurologic injury (including ICH, SAH, traumatic brain injury, and status epilepticus) benefit from standardized specialty care under the direction of a neurointensivist. Among stroke patients during the postacute inpatient phase, patients continue to be at risk for secondary neurologic injury such as cerebral edema, increased ICP, secondary or delayed ischemia and ischemic deficits, seizures, hydrocephalus, and fever-related injury, which are also time-sensitive emergencies. Neurointensivists have been shown to improve outcomes, LOS, and cost among neurocritically ill patients.[31–34] However, nationwide there are too few neurointensivists to provide on-site coverage for rapid assessment and treatment, particularly at night.[35] Telemedicine has been embraced as a strategy for improving safe and timely care to patients by allowing neurointensivists to have real-time access to patient information and bedside nurse inquires. As patients continue their recovery in the Neuro-ICU and throughout the care continuum, telemedicine also has a role in more chronic aspects of care for those who have incurred neurologic injury. The Telemedic Pilot Project for Integrative Stroke Care (TEMPiS) network in Bavaria and the Integrated Care for the Reduction of Secondary Stroke (ICARUSS) project in Australia are using telemedicine for follow-up of depressive symptoms in stroke survivors who return to the community.[36] Applying a telemedicine system for follow-up care in long-term facilities or at home to monitor therapy, functional mobility, and self-care status is conceivable.

The telestroke/teleneuro-ICU concept is compelling, but an important question is whether this system offers safe and effective stroke management. There has been a surge of telestroke projects in Europe and North America, which are accumulating evidence that stoke evaluation and treatment can safely and effectively be delivered via telestroke to centers without specialized stoke expertise routinely or immediately available (**Table 1**).[29] Feasibility and reliability of performing standardized clinical assessments by a stroke neurologist through videoconferencing with a bedside assistant has been shown in both nonacute and acute stroke settings.[37–44] Studies measuring the reliability of a neurologic examination by a telemedicine neurologist compared with face-to-face examination proved that it is reliable and satisfactory to the examiner and the patient.[45–47] In addition to physical examination, brain imaging with a noncontrast computed tomography (CT) scan is the crucial step to discerning the type of stroke (ischemic or hemorrhagic) and its chronicity. This assessment is mandatory before treatment with IV tPA. Although a neuroradiologist ideally interprets CT imaging, interpretation by a stroke neurologist in the absence of a neuroradiologist has been shown to be a safe substitute.[48,49] Three trials totaling 678 CT brain images of patients presenting with stroke symptoms found excellent agreement between a telestroke neurologist's and neuroradiologist's CT interpretation (sensitivity>87% for all feature except for hypodense basilar artery sign; specificity>98% for all features).[48–50] Feasibility, safety, and long-term outcomes of telestroke neurologists making treatment decisions have been supported in several open intervention studies.[23,38,51–53]

ESTABLISHING A TELESTROKE/NEUROLOGIC INTENSIVE CARE UNIT SYSTEM

Establishment of a telestroke or teleneuro-ICU system depends on the 2 main pillars of personnel and facility/technology development. A summary of requirements for both of these sectors is shown in **Table 2**. Setup for a telestroke and/or teleneuro-ICU program begins with a team of interested and engaged stroke neurologists and neurointensivists at a primary or comprehensive stroke center (hub) and regional hospitals (spokes) eager to collaborate with the hub team in the management of patients with strokes or who are neurocritically ill who arrive at the spoke facility. Although success relates to the efficiency and effectiveness of information transfer, there are a few major determinants of success of a telestroke/teleneuro-ICU program that are arguably more important than the telemedicine technology: (1) identifying willing and engaged stakeholders (champions) and relationship development between health care professionals in the facilities and throughout the network; (2) getting buy-in from referring physicians, administrative leadership, and telemedicine providers; (3) protocol development to standardize operations; (4) telemedicine education for all involved; and (5) developing a sustainability plan to keep hub and spoke partners engaged.[30] There are significant regulatory and legal barriers that must be overcome before setting up a telestroke network. A recent survey identified licensing out-of-state physicians, concern over malpractice liability, credentialing for medical staff privileges at individual institutions, and reimbursement limitations as major barriers to implementing and sustaining a telemedicine network.[54]

The selection of telecommunication and information technologies to provide real-time bidirectional audio and visual conferencing for stroke care is the next major step in the establishment of a telestroke/teleneuro-ICU program. The initial telemedicine system for stroke care, Telestroke 1.0, used a point-to-point model requiring consultants to travel to a workstation to provide consultations, which limited its usability and delayed treatment. This system was also limited to videoconferencing only.[50,55] In 1996, LaMonte and colleagues[56] developed a second-generation cellular phone technology (TeleBat project) that transmitted a photographic image every 2 seconds to a desktop. Although sending data over public wireless phone networks provided a low-cost, high-coverage, secure-transmission system, the low-bandwidth was technically challenging.

The ideal telestroke/teleneuro-ICU system is one that includes a high-quality, real-time, encrypted, audiovideo teleconferencing system; neuroimaging integration; mobility for site independence; decision and technical support features; electronic medical record integration; and billing and documentation that can be implemented across the World Wide Web.[55] At present, there are several telemedicine vendors that provide videoconferencing technology, integrated telestroke systems, and network services (including In Touch, Polycom, and Reach).[30] There are specific Centers for Medicare and Medicaid Services requirements for billing telestroke, which are highly influenced by the type of technology used, including (1) a high-quality 2-way video connection allowing the consultant to directly observe the patient while the patient, family, and clinicians view the consultant; (2) a video frame rate of 20 frames per second; (3) spoke bandwidth of at least 768 kbps to achieve minimal acceptable video quality; (4) camera controls that allow for point, tilt, and zoom functions for

Table 1
Evidence supporting assessment accuracy using telestroke

	Study	Study Design	Outcomes	Result
Video conference vs phone	Meyer et al,[101] 2008	Prospective RCT 111 to TS 111 to phone, n = 222	1. tPA treatment correct? 2. tPA use rate, ICH 3. 90 functional outcome	1. Correct treatment decision > with TM (98% TM vs 82% phone, P = .009) 2. No difference in other outcomes
	Demaerschalk et al,[102] 2010	Prospective RCT 22 to TS 24 to phone, n = 46	1. Treatment decision correct? 2. Rate tPA use 3. Mortality and ICH rate	No difference in outcomes between groups
NIHSS scoring reliability	Shafqat et al,[37] 1999	Comparative TS vs bedside, n = 20	1. NIHSS scoring time 2. Interrater reliability	1. TS score time longer than bedside (mean 9.7 vs 6.5 min, P<.001) 2. Strong correlation (r = 0.97, P<.001)
	Wang et al,[38] 2003	Comparative TS vs bedside, n= 20	NIHSS interrater correlation	Strong NIHSS score correlation between bedside and TS (r = 0.9552, P<.001)
	Handschu et al,[39] 2003	Comparative TS vs bedside, n = 41	1. NIHSS scoring time 2. Interrater reliability	1. TS score time longer (11.4 min vs 10.8 min, P<.013) 2. Excellent interrater agreement (kappa range 0.85–0.99)
	Meyer et al,[40] 2008	Comparative Naive-TS vs bedside, neurologist = 25	Interrater reliability for NIHSS and mRS	NIHSS: excellent interrater agreement (kappa = 0.974) mRS: excellent interrater agreement (kappa = 0.90)
	Meyer et al,[41] 2005	Comparative Wireless (laptop) TS vs bedside, n = 27	Interrater reliability	NIHSS: excellent interrater agreement (kappa = 0.94)
	Gonzalez et al,[42] 2011	Comparative Video phone vs n = 40 physicians, 480 paired comparisons	1. Time to perform sNIHSS 2. Method correlation and reliability	1. NIHSS examination 38 sec longer with video phone than bedside examination 2. Strong correlation between methods (r = 0.97, P<.01), high average reliability (0.99; 95% CI, 0.992–0.995)
	Anderson et al,[43] 2013	Comparative iPhone4 vs bedside, n = 20 patients	Interrater reliability	Excellent level of agreement (kappa = 0.98)
	Demaerschalk et al,[44] 2012	Comparative Smartphone vs bedside, n = 153 patients	Interrater reliability	Excellent NIHSS score correlation (r = 0.494; P<.001)

Neuro examination reliability	Craig et al,[45] 1999	Prospective reliability, n = 17	Feasibility and reliability of neuro examination with TM	1. Interobserver fair to perfect (k = 0.21–1.00) fair with eye movement
	Chua et al,[47] 2001	Prospective RCT F-F vs TM, n = 86	Satisfaction with TM	Satisfaction between methods except 2 domains Confidentiality concern with TM (P = .012) Embarrassment with TM (P = .005)
CT review reliability	Johnston et al,[48] 2003	Prospective reliability TS Neurologist and neuroradiologist, n = 72 images	Validity and reliability of neurologist's CT interpretation for ICH and HDS	Sensitivity (95% CI): 100% (0.93, 1.0) Specificity (95% CI): 100% (0.40, 0.98) Accuracy: 100% Kappa: 1.0
	Puetz et al,[49] 2013	Reliability/validity TS neurologist and neuroradiologist, n = 582 images	Validity and reliability of neurologist's CT interpretation	Sensitivity >87%, specificity >98% for ICH, tumor, hyperdense MCA, and dot sign Sensitivity 50%, specificity 98.8% for hyperdense basilar sign
	Demaerschalk et al,[103] 2012	RCT Phone: spoke/hub TS: telestroke/hub n = 54	Image agreement between neurologists using phone or TS with hub neuroradiologist	Phone: spoke/hub, >78% agreement for 6 features >68% agreement for chronic stroke TS/hub: >85% agreement for 5 features >73 for AIS, edema
	Schwamm et al,[50] 2004	Comparative Neurologist vs neuroradiologist, n = 24	1. Interrater reliability 2. User satisfaction	1. 100% agreement for imaging exclusion for tPA therapy 2. User endorsed VC for sound, image, connection speed, confidence managing patients

Abbreviations: AIS, acute ischemic stroke; F-F, face to face; MCA, middle cerebral artery; mRS, modified Rankin scale; NIHSS, National Institutes of Health Stroke Scale; RCT, randomized controlled trial; sNIHSS, simplified national institutes of health stroke scale; TM, telemedicine; TS, telestroke; VC, video conference.

Table 2
Personnel and facility requirements for establishing a telestroke or teleneuro ICU program

Personnel Requirements	Facilities Requirements
24/7 access to board-certified vascular neurologist (stroke specialist) and/or neurointensivist at telestroke/teleneuro-ICU center	Telemedicine computer and 2-way mobile camera including audio with user-friendly interfaces at requesting and consultant locations
Ability of consultant to be on camera within 15 min of initial consult	Encrypted telemedicine software, FDA/HIPAA compliant for continuous patient monitoring
Requesting physician who is educated on using telestroke/teleneuro-ICU equipment	High-speed Internet access
Nurse or licensed practitioner at requesting facility who can perform a neurologic examination, including the Glasgow Coma Scale and NIHSS	Image transfer connection between facilities to allow consultants to view brain imaging
Clear triggers at requesting facility for calling a telestroke or teleneuro-ICU consult	Ability to chart the consult and forward recommendations to requesting physician
Nurse trained in IV tPA administration	Ability to transfer the patient to a tertiary center if advanced stroke or neuro-ICU care is required (eg, angiography, neurosurgery, neuro-ICU monitoring)
Access to pharmacist or nurse to prepare tPA	Access to appropriate emergency medications, including IV tPA, blood pressure medications (eg, labetalol, nicardipine infusion, nimodipine), antiepileptics (eg, fosphenytoin, levetiracetam), coagulopathy reversal agents (eg, FFP, prothrombin, complex concentrates, protamine, vitamin K, cryoprecipitate), antifibrinolytics (eg, aminocaproic acid to prevent rebleed in aneurysmal subarachnoid hemorrhage), intracranial hypertension medications (eg, mannitol)
Technical support for maintenance troubleshooting	On-site and recurring training for the ED/hospital teams on both the referring and consultant sides
24/7 CT technologist who can perform emergency HCT and radiologist/neuro physician who can rapidly read and report head CT results	24/7 access to a CT scanner at the emergency facility

Abbreviations: ED, emergency department; FDA, food and drug administration; FFP, fresh frozen plasma; HCT, head computer tomography; HIPAA, health insurance portability and accountability act; ICU, intensive care unit; IV tPA, intravenous tissue plasminogen activator; NIHSS, national institutes of health stroke scale.

accurate remote National Institutes of Health Stroke Scale (NIHSS) assessment; (5) audio that is integrated into the video transmission or separately by telephone; and (6) remote neuroimaging (Digital Imaging and Communications in Medicine compatible) available to the consultant either integrated in the system or using a separate communication system with archiving capability.[30]

Robotic teledevices are also popular in some neuro-ICU and ED settings. Robotic telepresence (RTP) uses a robot that projects the image and voice of the intensivist through a flat screen and speakers mounted at the top of the robot. The robot moves around the ICU and ED controlled remotely by the intensivist or stroke neurologist.[57] This technology has proved to be a more efficient way for nurses to access help when needed rather than the paging and phone conversation paradigm. In a single-center prospective observational pre/post design, in which 2 neurointensivists rounded at night and responded to nursing pages using the RTP, there was a decrease in response time to face-to-face intensivist by 209 minutes, to brain ischemia alerts by 144 minutes, and to increased ICP alerts by 97 minutes (all $P<.001$). In addition, LOS was reduced by 1 to 2 days, ICU occupancy increased by 11%, and there was a cost saving of $1.1 million.[35] A second study at the same site using the robot was conducted to evaluate nursing satisfaction. Over a 4-week period, night nurses found the intensivist to be more available overall and present during acute emergencies ($P<.008$).[58] These results show promise that RTP can provide timely assessment and response to potential life-threatening brain injury in an intensive care setting.

WORKFLOW FOR TELESTROKE/TELENEUROLOGIC INTENSIVE CARE UNITS

The goal of using telestroke/teleneuro-ICU is to provide patients with timely expert neurologic evaluation, accurate treatment decisions, and a plan for further care and recovery at a facility equipped to meet the patient's needs. This time-sensitive process must be executed cooperatively and efficiently between the hub and spoke teams to optimize outcomes for patients. When a 911 call is dispatched to emergency medical services (EMS), it is important that both primary and comprehensive stroke centers and spoke facilities participating in telestroke/teleneuro-ICU networks can be identified by the EMS team. Optimally, stroke or strokelike symptoms/signs are identified by EMS and prehospital notification to the ED occurs. Before EMS arrival, a stroke alert should have prepared the ED for the patient's arrival. The clinical team must then be prepared to begin initial brain protection care immediately and initiate a telestroke or tele-ICU consultation for further management guidance. Typical consult triggers are listed in **Box 2**. After remote access to the patient and spoke hospital team has been established, the telestroke neurologist gathers a brief but comprehensive history from the patient or representative, performs a neurologic examination (NIHSS) with the bedside nurse, reviews the head CT with the spoke physician, and provides treatment in collaboration with the spoke physician. There are established door-to-goal times for each element of care, particularly refined for delivering tPA in the optimal time frame of less than 60 minutes from door to needle. A flow path for telestroke/teleneuro-ICU is shown in **Fig. 1**.

Box 2
Triggers for telestroke or teleneuro-ICU consult
Triggers
Sudden weakness or focal deficits
Sudden language problem
Sudden facial weakness
Sudden dysarthria
New difficulty ambulating
Severe headache and/or neck stiffness
Loss of consciousness or coma
Seizurelike activity

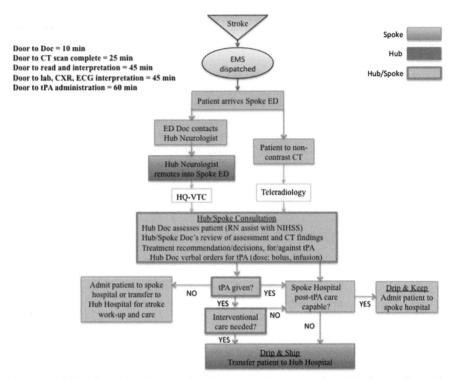

Fig. 1. Workflow for telestroke consults. CT, computed tomography; CXR, chest radiograph; Doc, doctor; ECG, electrocardiogram; ED, emergency department; EMS, emergency medical service; NIHSS, national institute of health stroke scale; tPA, tissue plasminogen activator.

The American Heart Association/American Stroke Association has released a guideline with recommendations for the implementation of telemedicine within stroke systems of care (**Table 3**).[4,7]

ACUTE MANAGEMENT OF PATIENTS IN TELESTROKE/NEUROLOGIC INTENSIVE CARE UNITS

There are many types of neurologic emergency that can be efficiently handled via telemedicine. The most common are ischemic stroke, hemorrhagic stroke, traumatic brain injury, and seizures. A brief overview of the emergency management of each of these disorders is presented later. A critical first step when a patient presents with neurologic symptoms is to obtain an accurate history, including the time last known normal (not the time the patient was found with symptoms) followed by a targeted neurologic examination. The NIHSS developed for use in acute stroke therapy trials and the Glasgow Coma Score are commonly used standardized neurologic assessments.[59,60] After stabilization, including assessment for the need for intubation, establishment of IV access, and maintenance of adequate blood pressure (mean arterial pressure ≥65 mm Hg), noncontrast head CT imaging should be performed. If stroke is suspected, the recommended time from door to CT scan is 25 minutes. Based on the head CT findings and history, the telestroke/teleneuro-ICU physician embarks on different acute management paradigms, as discussed later.

Table 3
American Heart Association and American Stroke Association scientific statement on use of telemedicine in patients with suspected acute ischemic stroke

Recommendation	Grade of Recommendation	Level of Evidence
NIHSS examination performed	Class I	A
NIHSS examination by stroke specialist: acute setting	Class I	A
General neurologic examination performed	Class IIa	B
Teleradiology system approved by FDA or similar governing body for:		
Timely review of CT scan	Class I	B
Review of brain CT scans by stroke specialist	Class I	A
Rapid image interpretation in time for tPA decision making	Class I	B
Medical opinion in favor or against use of IV tPA provided by stroke specialist	Class I	B
Consultation in conjunction with stroke education and training for health care providers to improve use of IV tPA at community hospitals without stroke expertise	Class II	B
Telephone consultation for safely and effectively administering IV tPA	Class IIb	C
Telephone-based communication between EMS personnel and stroke specialist for enrollment in hyperacute neuroprotective trials	Class IIa	B
Inpatient stroke consultation when local stroke expertise unavailable	Class I	B
Assessment of physical, occupational, speech disability by allied health profession using specific assessments when in-person assessment impractical	Class I	B
Telephone assessment for measuring functional disability after stroke, when in-person assessment not available, using rating scales validated for phone using structured interview by trained personnel	Class I	B

Abbreviations: CT, computed tomography; EMS, emergency medical service; FDA, food and drug administration; IV tPA, intravenous tissue plasminogen activator; NIHSS, national institutes of health stroke scale.

Acute Ischemic Stroke Management

A major breakthrough for stroke treatment came with the landmark National Institute of Neurological Disorders and Stroke rt-TPA Stroke Study Group (NINDS) trial, which showed that patients treated with IV tPA less than 3 hours after an acute ischemic stroke were 30% more likely to have complete to near-complete neurologic recovery at 3 months compared with patients not treated with tPA.[10] Shortly after this trial, IV tPA was approved by the US Food and Drug Administration (FDA) and remains the only FDA-approved treatment of acute ischemic stroke to improve neurologic recovery and functional outcomes.[61] Several studies have investigated the safety of tPA, but the most convincing data come from the Safe Implementation of Thrombolysis in Stroke–International Stroke Thrombolysis Register (SITS-ISTR). From this registry of 11,865 patients treated with IV tPA within 3 hours of stroke symptom onset, the frequency of symptomatic ICH was 1.6% (95% confidence interval [CI], 1.4%–1.8%) and favorable outcomes (modified Rankin scale [mRS], 0, 1, 2) at 90 days occurred in 56% (95% CI, 55.3%–57.2%).[62] Subsequently, 2 trials investigating the safety and benefit of IV tPA therapy in patients greater than 80 years old showed comparable outcomes with patients of younger age.[3,63] In addition, Lyerly and colleagues[64] showed that patients with prior infarcts on CT scan did not experience more symptomatic ICH (4% vs 2%; P = .221) or hemorrhagic transformation (18% vs 14%; P = .471). The European Cooperative Acute Stroke Study (ECASS) III showed that the window of opportunity for treating acute ischemic stroke with IV tPA could be extended to 4.5 hours.[65] Although efficacious out to 4.5 hours, IV tPA is most beneficial when given within the first 90 minutes for restoring blood flow and preserving functional outcome. An analysis of pooled trials (N = 3696) evaluating the impact of onset time to tPA treatment on 3-month outcomes found that the odds of a favorable 3-month outcome (function and mortality) increased as time to treatment decreased (P = .03), and it was concluded that the odds of a favorable outcome are greatest when tPA is given within 90 minutes of stroke symptom onset, but benefit exists out to 4.5 hours from ictus (**Fig. 2**). Thus, the narrow window for effective intervention with IV tPA makes this therapy extremely time sensitive. Inclusion and exclusion criteria for the administration of IV tPA are listed in **Table 4**.

Although the benefits of tPA have been well shown in several safety and efficacy studies, there are risks to this treatment, which need to be communicated to the patient and/or patient representative (**Table 5**). However, IV tPA is standard of care and consent is not required for administration, although disclosure of the benefits and risks is suggested before administration. Dosing tPA is based on the patient's weight in kilograms. A total dose of 0.9 mg/kg (maximum 90 mg) is divided with 10% given as an

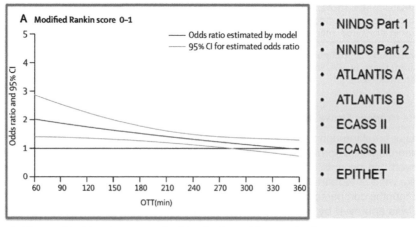

Fig. 2. Time to IV tPA treatment and odds of a favorable neurologic outcome at 3 months. ATLANTIS, alteplace thrombolysis for acute nonintervenal therapy in ischemic stroke; ECASS, european cooperative acute stroke study; EPITHET, ecoplanar imaging thrombolytic evaluation trial; NINDS, national institutes of neurological disorders and stroke; OTT, onset to treatment. (*From* Lees KR, Bluhmki E, von Kummer R, et al. Time to treatment with intravenous alteplase and outcome in stroke: an updated pooled analysis of ECASS, ATLANTIS, NINDS, and EPITHET trials. Lancet 2010;375(9727):1699; with permission.)

Table 4 Inclusion and exclusion criteria for administering IV rt-tPA	
Inclusion ≤3 h and ≤3–4.5	• Diagnosis of ischemic stroke causing measurable neurologic deficit • Witnessed onset of symptoms or last known normal ≤3 h or <3–4.5 h before beginning treatment • Age ≥18 y
Exclusion ≤3 h and ≤3–4.5 h	• Significant head trauma or prior stroke in previous 3 mo • Symptoms suggest SAH • Arterial puncture at noncompressible site in previous 7 d • History of ICH • Intracranial neoplasm, arteriovenous malformation, or aneurysm • Recent intracranial or intraspinal surgery • Increased blood pressure (systolic>185 mm Hg or diastolic>110 mm Hg) • Active internal bleeding • Acute bleeding diathesis, including but not limited to platelet count <100,000/mm³ • Heparin received within 48 h, resulting in abnormally increased aPTT greater than the upper limit of normal • Current use of anticoagulant with INR>1.7 or PT>15 sec • Current use of direct thrombin inhibitors or direct factor Xa inhibitors (rivaroxaban, dabigatran, apixaban) with increased sensitive laboratory tests (such as aPTT, INR, platelet count, and ECT, TT, or appropriate factor Xa activity assays) • Blood glucose concentration <50 mg/dL (2.7 mmol/L) • CT shows multilobar infarction (hypodensity>one-third cerebral hemisphere) Relative exclusion criteria: • Only minor or rapidly improving stroke symptoms (clearing spontaneously) • Pregnancy • Seizure at onset with postictal residual neurologic impairments • Major surgery or serious trauma within previous 14 d • Recent gastrointestinal or urinary tract hemorrhage (within previous 21 d) • Recent acute myocardial infarction (within previous 3 mo)
Additional exclusion for ≤3–4.5 h	• Age>80 y • Severe stroke (NIHSS>25) • Taking an oral anticoagulant regardless of INR • History of both diabetes and prior ischemic stroke

Abbreviations: aPTT, activated partial thromboplastin time; d, day; ECT, ecarin clotting time; h, hour; INR, international normalized ratio; mm Hg, millimeters mercury; mo, month; NIHSS, national institutes of health stroke scale; PT, prothrombin time; TT, thrombin time.

initial bolus over 1 minute and the remaining 90% is given as an infusion over 60 minutes. Because higher doses of tPA (1.0 mg/kg) have not shown benefit and impose a higher risk of hemorrhagic conversion, it is mandatory that patients be weighed accurately before IV tPA administration. Inclusion for tPA therapy requires the patient's blood pressure to be less than 185/110 mm Hg. Blood pressure–reducing agents such as IV labetalol, hydralazine, or enalaprilat, and/or nicardipine infusion to control blood pressure, can be used (**Table 6**). Although some guidelines suggest the use of nitroprusside for refractory blood pressure increases, we do not endorse its use because it is known to increase ICP.[66]

Table 5
Risks and benefits of IV tPA therapy

	≤3 h	3–4.5 h
Benefits	13% chance of being left with minimal or no disability (mRS 0–1)	7% chance of being left with minimal or no disability (mRS 0–1)
	1 more patient out of every 7.7 patients left with minimal or no disability (mRS 0–1)	1 more patient out of every 14 patients left with minimal or no disability (mRS 0–1)
	1 in 3 patients improve by at least 1 grade in the mRS	1 in 6.25 patients improve by at least 1 grade in the mRS
	Global odds ratio for favorable outcome 1.7 (95% CI 1.2–2.6)	
Risks	6.4% incidence of symptomatic ICH within 36 h (~10× increased risk)	7.9% incidence of symptomatic ICH within 36 h (~2× increased risk)
	1 in 32 patients have a worsening of at least 1 grade in the mRS	1 in 37 patients have a worsening of at least 1 grade in the mRS
	Angioedema: Occurs in <1% of stroke cases treated with tPA[95]	
	Symptoms: swelling of lips, tongue, oropharynx. May be mild, can be severe	
	Particularly associated with ACE inhibitor and β-blocker (less so) use	
	Monitoring parameters: check patient for symptoms at 45, 60, 75 min after tPA	
	Treatment:	
	Diphenhydramine (Benadryl) 50 mg IV; ranitidine (Zantac) 50 mg IV	
	Methylprednisolone (Solu-Medrol) 50–100 mg IV; racemic epinephrine	
	Monitor for intubation	

Abbreviation: ACE, angiotensin-converting enzyme.

Data from Tissue plasminogen activator for acute ischemic stroke. The National Institute Of Neurological Disorders and Stroke rt-PA Stroke Study Group. N Engl J Med 1995;333(24):1581–7.

Table 6
Monitoring and blood pressure management before, during, and after tPA

Vital signs	q 15 min × 2 h from start of IV tPA
	Then q 30 min × 6 h
	Then q 60 min × 16 h for total of 24 h of close vital signs and neuro checks
	Then vital signs and neuro checks per physician order

BP Goal (mm Hg)	BP Range (mm Hg)	BP Management
Pre-tPA<185/110	BP>185/110	Labetalol 10–20 mg IV over 1–2 min; may repeat 1 time
		Or
		Nicardipine 5 mg/h IV, titrate up to 2.5 mg/h every 1–15 min; maximum 15 mg/h[a]
Intra-tPA, post-tPA <180/105	Systolic>180–230 Or Diastolic 105–120	Labetalol 10 mg IV push followed by infusion at 2–8 mg/min
		Or
		Nicardipine 5 mg/h IV, titrate up to 2.5 mg/h every 1–15 min, maximum 15 mg/h
	BP not controlled or diastolic>140 mm Hg	Combination of labetalol and nicardipine infusion

Abbreviation: BP, blood pressure.

  [a] Hydralazine or enalaprilat can be used.

Data from Schwamm LH, Holloway RG, Amarenco P, et al. A review of the evidence for the use of telemedicine within stroke systems of care: a scientific statement from the American Heart Association/American Stroke Association. Stroke 2009;40(7):2616–34; and Jauch EC, Saver JL, Adams HP, Jr, et al. Guidelines for the early management of patients with acute ischemic stroke: a guideline for healthcare professionals from the American Heart Association/American Stroke Association. Stroke 2013;44(3):870–947.

Patients with high NIHSS scores suggesting large-vessel occlusion, or those that show large-vessel occlusion on imaging (such as CT or magnetic resonance angiography) may be candidates for IA therapy such as IA tPA or mechanical clot retrieval. Typical time windows for endovascular treatment include less than or equal to 6 hours from ictus for IA tPA and less than or equal to 8 hours from ictus for clot retrieval. In certain circumstances, such as posterior circulation stroke or in cases of MRI diffusion/perfusion mismatch, this window can be extended. It is essential that telestroke programs develop a relationship with treatment centers that offer endovascular management options.

The major risk of IV tPA use is symptomatic ICH (sICH), occurring in 5% to 6.4% of patients most commonly within the first 24 hours after tPA is administered.[10,67] Symptoms include headache, decrease in mental status, worsening neurologic symptoms, increase in blood pressure and pulse, nausea, and vomiting. If ICH is suspected, IV tPA infusion should be stopped and immediate noncontrast head CT should be performed along with simultaneous blood draw for prothrombin time (PT), partial thromboplastin time (PTT), International Normalized Ratio (INR), and fibrinogen. Administering cryoprecipitate (10 units) to restore depleted fibrinogen stores is recommended.[62,68,69] In patients who cannot tolerate cryoprecipitate transfusion, antifibrinolytics such as tranexamic acid or aminocaproic acid may be considered.[70] Reducing the blood pressure to a systolic goal of less than 140 mm Hg to prevent ICH expansion is also recommended.[71] If hemorrhagic conversion or hemorrhage related to tPA is detected, transfer to a neurocritical care ICU setting is recommended.

Hemorrhagic Stroke (Subarachnoid Hemorrhage and Intracerebral Hemorrhagic Stroke) Management

Intracerebral hemorrhagic stroke (ICH) and cerebral aneurysm rupture causing SAH account for 8% to 15% and 3% of all stroke types, respectively.[72–74] Both ICH and SAH are severe illnesses that carry mortalities as high as 50% in the first month.[75–77] The 30-day mortalities for ICH range from 35% to 50%.[73,75,78] and up to 50% of these patients die within the first 2 days.[79] Between 12% and 39% of patients with ICH achieve functional independence.[78] Among patients with SAH, 12% die before reaching the hospital, 12% are misdiagnosed in the ED, 25% die in the hospital, and 30-day mortality is 45%.[77,80,81] Up to 40% of patients with SAH are unable to return to work and nearly 60% experience psychological sequelae including depression.[82,83] Despite historically catastrophic outcomes, many patients with hemorrhagic stroke improve substantially and return to a high quality of life with early aggressive medical, surgical, and endovascular interventions.

Blood pressure management, coagulopathy reversal, and treatment of symptoms of increased ICP are critical to early management of ICH. ICH expansion occurs in approximately 38% of patients with ICH within the first 3 hours of onset.[84] Similarly, aneurysm rerupture in patients with SAH is most common within the first day of initial rupture. The first-line intervention for preventing hematoma expansion or aneurysm rerupture is reducing the systolic blood pressure to less than 140 mm Hg with nicardipine infusion (5–15 mg/h IV) or labetalol (20 mg IV push or infusion at 2 mg/min) as first-line agents.[71,85,86] Nitroprusside and nitroglycerin should be avoided because of the risk of labile blood pressure and increased ICP.[71] In patients with SAH, antifibrinolytics such as aminocaproic acid and tranexamic acid have been shown to reduce rebleed rates from 7% to 2% when administered within 72 hours of ictus.[14]

Coagulopathy reversal should be considered for all patients with ICH. Coagulopathy can be caused by pharmacologic therapy and/or intrinsic processes such as thrombocytopenia, end-stage renal disease, or liver failure. Indications for coagulopathy reversal include[86,87]:

- Increased PTT or INR greater than 1.4 caused by the disease process or pharmacologically induced.
- Warfarin therapy: regardless of the size of the ICH or the indication for antithrombotic therapy, reversal should occur. Reversal can be considered in patients with normal INR in select circumstances (eg, the patient has just started warfarin and the INR may not reflect the patient's true coagulopathic state).
- tPA therapy: for all patients who received tPA 24 hours before ICH regardless of size or symptoms of ICH.
- Antiplatelet use (aspirin, clopidogrel, or other adenosine diphosphate (ADP) inhibitors): platelet transfusion is recommended only if the agent was taken within the last 7 days and patient is undergoing neurosurgical procedure. DDAVP (desmopressin [1-desamino-8-D-arginine vasopressin]; 0.4 µg/kg IV × 1) may be given to improve global hemostasis in patients with antiplatelet-associated ICH.
- Fondaparinux, danaparoid, dalteparin, tinzaparin, dabigatran, bivalirudin, argatroban, apixaban, or rivaroxaban therapy: there are few data supporting the efficacy of reversal agents.
- Other considerations: patients receiving anticoagulation with known cerebral sinus thrombosis should not undergo coagulopathy reversal even in the context of ICH. In patients with acute, severe concomitant thrombosis (ie, large acute myocardial infarction or pulmonary embolus with hemodynamic instability), risks versus benefits of coagulopathy reversal should be carefully weighed on a patient-by-patient basis.

Coagulopathy reversal recommendations are shown in **Table 7**.

Increased ICP is a life-threatening complication of ICH. Rapid progression of cerebral edema followed by increasing ICP and brain herniation can precipitate rapid neurologic deterioration and further brain injury. Early warning signs of increasing ICP include drowsiness, headache, visual disturbance, disconjugate gaze, nausea, vomiting, and unilateral dilated pupil.[88]

There are several measures to be taken to reduce ICP, including upright head positioning to improve venous return, hyperventilation for temporary vasoconstriction, hyperosmolar therapy to decrease edema, and external ventricular drain to divert cerebral spinal fluid, and these measures are outlined in **Fig. 3**. Because all patients with SAH and some patients with ICH require surgical or endovascular intervention, it is essential that, after acute teleneuro-ICU stabilization, such patients be transferred to tertiary facilities that are staffed by experienced neurosurgeons, neurointerventionalists, and neurointensivists.

Traumatic Brain Injury Management

Patients with traumatic brain injury develop brain contusions, intracerebral hemorrhage, subdural and epidural hematomas, and diffuse cerebral edema. These patients may have concomitant skull and spine fractures that require neurosurgical intervention. Similar to patients with ICH, acute telemedicine management of patients with traumatic brain injury consists of coagulopathy reversal, blood pressure management, and treatment of increased ICP in a fashion similar to that delineated earlier. Because hypoxia and hypotension are major predictors of poor outcome after traumatic brain injury, these complications should be managed aggressively. Cervical spine

Table 7
Coagulopathy reversal in patients with ICH

Warfarin	• Vitamin K 10 mg IV × 1 • PCC 10–50 units/kg depending on type of PCC and INR or FFP 10–15 mL/kg
Apixaban, dabigatran, rivaroxaban	• FEIBA 50 units/kg × 1 • Consider activated charcoal with ingestion of apixaban or rivaroxaban within 2 h • Consider hemodialysis for dabigatran, particularly in patients with underlying renal insufficiency
Antiplatelet (aspirin, Aggrenox, abciximab eptifibatide, tirofiban, clopidogrel, prasugrel, ticagrelor use in last 3 d)	• 1–2 apheresis unit platelets for patients undergoing a neurosurgical procedure Do not transfuse platelets unless neurosurgical procedure is planned • Antiplatelet use or von Willebrand disease: DDAVP 0.4 μg/kg × 1 (20 μg in 50 mL NS over 15–30 min)
Thrombocytopenia	• Transfuse for platelet count <50,000/mm³
End-stage renal disease	• DDAVP 0.4 μg/kg × 1 (20 μg in 50 mL NS over 15–30 min) + 1 apheresis unit platelets
Liver disease with known coagulopathy or increased PT or INR ≥1.5	1. Vitamin K 10 mg IV over 10 min (monitor for hypotension/anaphylaxis) and 2. PCC 10–50 units/kg depending on type of PCC and INR 3. If INR ≥2.0, give 10–15 mL/kg of FFP 4. If PCC unavailable, 10–15 mL/kg of FFP total
Unfractionated heparin (enoxaparin; protamine has negligible effect on danaparoid or fondaparinux)	• Continuous infusion: calculate the total dose the patient received during the last 2.5 h, then dose protamine 1.0 mg per 100 units of heparin (eg, 1200 U/h × 2.5 h = 3000 U; at 1.0 mg/100 U = 30 mg protamine) • If a bolus of heparin was given within the last 30 min, the bolus dose should be reversed at 1.0 mg protamine per 100 U heparin • If a bolus of heparin was given 31–60 min prior, 0.5 mg protamine per 100 U heparin should be given • Protamine: maximum dose 50 mg; no more than 50 mg should be given over any 10-min period; monitor for anaphylaxis and hypotension

Low-molecular-weight heparin	• Enoxaparin (Lovenox): 1 mg protamine IV per 1 mg of enoxaparin given in last 8 h:
	  1. If 8–12 h since enoxaparin dosed, 0.5 mg protamine IV per 1 mg of enoxaparin
	  2. If bleeding continues and/or aPTT is prolonged 2–4 h after first dose of protamine: 0.5 mg protamine IV per 1 mg of enoxaparin
	  3. If >12 h since last dose of enoxaparin, no protamine
	• Protamine has negligible reversal effects on danaparoid and fondaparinux. Consider FFP, PCC, or rVIIa
	• Dalteparin or tinzaparin: 1 mg protamine for each 100 anti-Xa IU of dalteparin or tinzaparin;
	• If bleeding, consider additional dose of 0.5 mg for each 100 anti-Xa IU of dalteparin or tinzaparin

tPA (alteplase, reteplase, tenecteplase)	• Cryoprecipitate 10 units

Abbreviations: DDAVP, desmopressin (1-desamino-8-D-arginine vasopressin); FEIBA, factor 8 inhibitor bypassing activity; FFP, fresh frozen plasma; INR, international normalizing ratio; IU, international units; IV, intravenous; NS, normal saline; PCC, prothrombin complex concentrates; rVIIa, recombinant factor 7 activated; tPA, tissue plasminogen activator; U, units.

Data from Morgenstern LB, Hemphill JC, 3rd, Anderson C, et al. Guidelines for the management of spontaneous intracerebral hemorrhage: a guideline for healthcare professionals from the American Heart Association/American Stroke Association. Stroke 2010;41(9):2108–29; and Andrews CM, Jauch EC, Hemphill JC,3rd, Smith WS, Weingart SD. Emergency neurological life support: intracerebral hemorrhage. Neurocrit Care 2012;17(Suppl 1):S37–46.

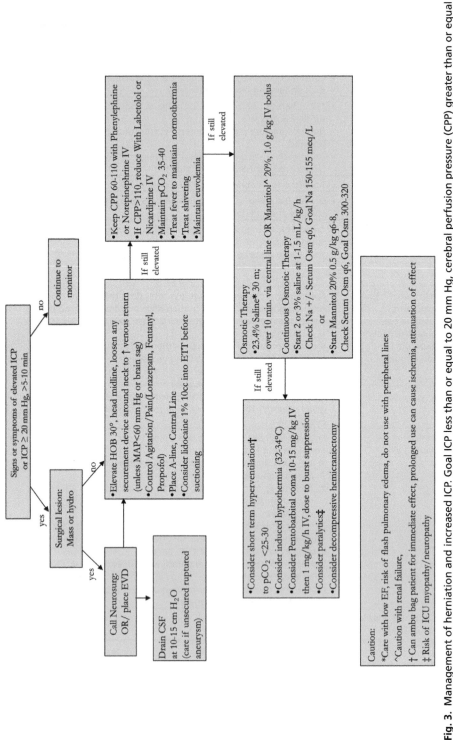

Fig. 3. Management of herniation and increased ICP. Goal ICP less than or equal to 20 mm Hg, cerebral perfusion pressure (CPP) greater than or equal to 60 mm Hg. CSF, cerebrospinal fluid; EF, ejection fraction; ETT, endotracheal tube; EVD, external ventricular drain; HOB, head of bed; MAP, mean arterial pressure.

immobilization and imaging (noncontrast cervical spine CT) may be indicated as well. As with patients with SAH and ICH, transfer to a tertiary facility equipped to treat head trauma is indicated.

Seizure Management

Specific interventions for seizure treatment are outlined in **Table 8**.

POSTTELESTROKE/TELENEUROLOGIC INTENSIVE CARE UNIT CARE

The final step in telestroke or teleneuro-ICU consultation is determining the best facility for the patient to receive further care. Critical factors for deciding disposition include the need for neurosurgical or endovascular intervention for further evaluation and treatment, access to continuous electroencephalogram monitoring, and the level of neurocritical care required. Neurocritical illness severity and the spoke hospital's resources factor heavily in this decision, because hospitals with dedicated stroke and neurocritical care ICUs that care for high volumes of severe stroke, SAH, and ICH have been shown to improve outcomes.[31–33,62,86,89] Primary or comprehensive stroke care accreditation markedly improves the delivery of organized, systematic, efficient stroke care that is evidence based and universally accepted and practiced.[90] Four separate studies found that treating critically ill patients with neurologic injury in a neurocritical care specialty ICU staffed by neurointensivists and neurologically trained nurses favorably altered clinical outcomes.[31–34] A neurointensivist-staffed ICU significantly reduced the risk of death by 42% during the first 3 days of neonatal ICU stay ($P \leq .003$)[34] and is associated with lower overall mortalities (odds ratio, 0.388; 95% CI, 0.22–0.67).[31] In addition, admission into an

Table 8	
Teleneuro-ICU seizure management paradigm	
First-line agent	Check blood glucose. Administer thiamine followed by D50 if glucose low or unknown
	Lorazepam IV (0.1 mg/kg maximum dose), in 2-mg or 4-mg IV aliquots until seizure termination[104–106]
Second-line agent	Fosphenytoin 20 mg/kg IV loading dose. Fosphenytoin can be given at a maximum rate of 150 mg/min (infusion rate 20–30 min on average). A slower rate is acceptable, and is recommended for the elderly, those with relative hypotension, and those at risk of cardiac arrhythmias
Third-line agent	In patients who continue to seize after fosphenytoin load or those with seizures >5 min in duration, immediate intubation should occur followed by midazolam drip (0.2 mg/kg IV bolus, then 0.2–2.0 mg/kg/h)
Ongoing monitoring and management	Continuous EEG monitoring is indicated for patients with depressed mental status out of proportion to the degree of brain injury
	Recommend 24 h of continuous EEG monitoring in noncomatose patients and 48 h of BEM in comatose patients[107]
	If no continuous EEG monitoring at spoke hospital, transfer patient to facility with continuous EEG monitoring
	Evaluation for seizure cause may include checking antiepileptic drug levels (if patient has a history of seizure on medication), MRI with contrast, lumbar puncture, toxicology screen

Abbreviations: BEM, bedside electroencephalogram monitoring; EEG, electroencephalogram; ICU, intensive care unit.

established neuro-ICU is associated with decreased ICU and hospital LOS (both $P<.0001$)[32] and improved discharge disposition.[34] In addition, total costs of care are lower than the national benchmark in neuro-ICUs run by neuro intensivists ($P<.01$).[33]

THE NEXT FRONTIER: MOBILE STROKE TREATMENT UNITS

Even though telemedicine has been proved to increase access to the delivery of tPA to patients who have had strokes, symptom onset to treatment time has stalled at an average of 132 minutes.[10,23,53,55,91–95] Delivery of tPA also remains extremely low at 2% to 7%.[19] The greatest time delay is during the prehospital phase, which has widely been unaffected by advancements in stroke care.[96] As telemedicine capabilities evolve and evidence builds supporting telestroke as a safe, accurate, and efficient system for providing stroke care, bold new approaches are being taken to reach patients sooner. Instead of immediate transport to an ED, delivering the stroke team, point-of-care diagnostics, portable CT scanner, clinical stroke physician via telemedicine technology, and pharmacologic treatments to the patient in a disease-specific ambulance prompted the development of the mobile stroke unit (MSU).[19,27,97] First developed in Germany, the MSU has improved both onset-to-treatment times and the rate of tPA delivery.[19,27,97]

The impetus for creating an MSU was the realization that combating the devastation of stroke and the poststroke cost burden will not be met until stroke care starts at the prehospital phase. The goal of the MSU is to reach stroke patients early, bring the highest level of care to patients as fast as possible, and to achieve a benchmark of less than 60 minutes for evaluation and treatment of tPA. The concept of an MSU was first realized in Homburg, Germany, under the direction of Klaus Fassbender, then by the Stroke Emergency Mobile (STEMO) project in Berlin, Germany, in 2008.[27,92] This project has shown feasibility, safety, and efficiency in dramatically shortening time to stroke diagnosis and treatment.[91,92,98] The Prehospital Acute Neurological Treatment and Optimization of Medical Care in Stroke Study (PHAN-TOM-S) randomized patients to MSU care versus standard EMS care in 5282 subjects (3213 STEMO group, 2969 control group). The time from notification to stroke treatment was significantly reduced in the MSU group compared with the control group by 25 minutes (95% CI, 20–29 minutes; $P<.001$). In addition, the rate of thrombolysis

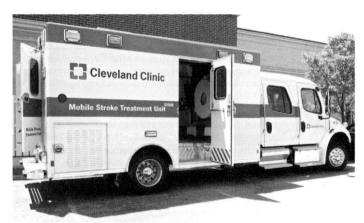

Fig. 4. MSU. Note that the CereTom CT scanner and diagnostic laboratory are located in the back of the ambulance.

treatment of the MSU group was 33% versus 21% in the control group (12% difference; 95% CI, 7–16; P<.001). There were no differences in tPA-associated ICH rates or 7-day mortality.[92] These exceptional results reinforce that starting care at the prehospital phase is the right model for safe, efficient, and effective stroke care delivery. This strategy also creates an opportunity to provide patients with early cause-specific therapies such as blood pressure management for ischemic stroke (higher blood pressure goals) versus hemorrhagic stroke (lower blood pressure goals)[71] and organized, accurate triage to the most appropriate hospital based on diagnosis clarified before transport.

MSUs exist in two German sites (Berlin and Homburg). In the United States, a MSU was created at the University of Texas Health Science Center in Houston, Texas (UTHealth) and a Mobile Stroke Treatment Unit (MSTU) was created at Cleveland Clinic Foundation in Cleveland, Ohio. These units are equipped with a CT scanner, point-of-care laboratory, telecommunication for transfer of imaging (teleradiology), and videoconferencing for stroke expert consultation support. The units are staffed with a nurse, paramedic, and CT technologist and emergency

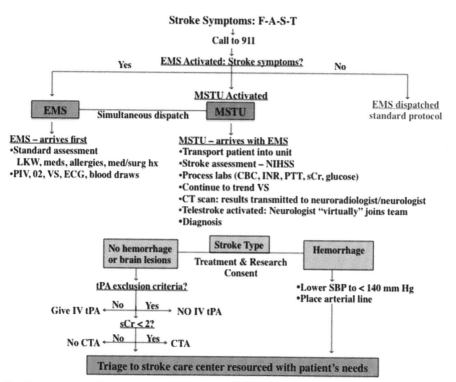

Fig. 5. MSTU workflow. F-A-S-T stroke symptoms include face weakness, arm weakness, speech abnormalities or slurring, and time (acute onset). CBC, complete blood count; CTA, CT angiography; LKW, last known well; NIHSS, NIH stroke scale; PIV, peripheral IV; SBP, systolic blood pressure; sCr, serum creatinine; VS, vital signs. (*Data from* Kothari RU, Pancioli A, Liu T, et al. Cincinnati prehospital stroke scale: reproducibility and validity. Ann Emerg Med 1999;33(4):373–8; and Studnek JR, Asimos A, Dodds J, et al. Assessing the validity of the Cincinnati Prehospital Stroke Scale and the Medic Prehospital Assessment for Code Stroke in an urban emergency medical services agency. Prehosp Emerg Care 2013; 17(3):348–53.)

medical technician. The German and UTHealth units have a neurologist on board.[99,100] Cleveland Clinic's MSTU model brings the stroke neurologist virtually into the unit using telestroke technology. This briefcase-sized telemedicine unit uses encrypted mobile broadband links that allow both rapid transfer of CT scan images and videoconferencing with a stroke neurologist from Cleveland Clinic's comprehensive stroke center (**Fig. 4**). The workflow of a MSTU differs from standard telemedicine and is outlined in **Fig. 5**.

SUMMARY

With advancements in information and communication technologies, telestroke and teleneuro-ICU are now part of mainstream clinical practice and are safe, reliable, cost-saving strategies that improve the timely response to neuro-ICU emergencies, decrease hospital LOS, and improved functional outcomes.[35,36,52,99] Telestroke reduces disparities in access to expert care, ensuring that no hospital remains underserved and no patients with acute stroke receive suboptimal care.[27] The next frontier in telestroke/teleneuro-ICU involves MSTUs that can further shorten the time to diagnosis and treatment.

REFERENCES

1. Marini C, Baldassarre M, Russo T, et al. Burden of first-ever ischemic stroke in the oldest old: evidence from a population-based study. Neurology 2004; 62(1):77–81.
2. Di Carlo A, Baldereschi M, Gandolfo C, et al. Stroke in an elderly population: incidence and impact on survival and daily function. The Italian Longitudinal Study on Aging. Cerebrovasc Dis 2003;16(2):141–50.
3. Mishra NK, Ahmed N, Andersen G, et al. Thrombolysis in very elderly people: controlled comparison of SITS International Stroke Thrombolysis Registry and Virtual International Stroke Trials Archive. BMJ 2010;341:c6046.
4. Schwamm LH, Holloway RG, Amarenco P, et al. A review of the evidence for the use of telemedicine within stroke systems of care: a scientific statement from the American Heart Association/American Stroke Association. Stroke 2009;40(7): 2616–34.
5. Johnston SC, Mendis S, Mathers CD. Global variation in stroke burden and mortality: estimates from monitoring, surveillance, and modelling. Lancet Neurol 2009;8(4):345–54.
6. Go AS, Mozaffarian D, Roger VL, et al. Heart disease and stroke statistics–2014 update: a report from the American Heart Association. Circulation 2014;129(3): e28–292.
7. Schwamm LH, Audebert HJ, Amarenco P, et al. Recommendations for the implementation of telemedicine within stroke systems of care: a policy statement from the American Heart Association. Stroke 2009;40(7):2635–60.
8. Brown DL, Boden-Albala B, Langa KM, et al. Projected costs of ischemic stroke in the United States. Neurology 2006;67(8):1390–5.
9. Rosamond W, Flegal K, Furie K, et al. Heart disease and stroke statistics–2008 update: a report from the American Heart Association Statistics Committee and Stroke Statistics Subcommittee. Circulation 2008;117(4):e25–146.
10. Tissue plasminogen activator for acute ischemic stroke. the national institute of neurological disorders and stroke rt-PA stroke study group. N Engl J Med 1995; 333(24):1581–7.

11. Vahedi K, Hofmeijer J, Juettler E, et al. Early decompressive surgery in malignant infarction of the middle cerebral artery: a pooled analysis of three randomised controlled trials. Lancet Neurol 2007;6(3):215–22.
12. Saver JL. Time is brain–quantified. Stroke 2006;37(1):263–6.
13. Naidech AM, Janjua N, Kreiter KT, et al. Predictors and impact of aneurysm rebleeding after subarachnoid hemorrhage. Arch Neurol 2005;62(3):410–6.
14. Hillman J, Fridriksson S, Nilsson O, et al. Immediate administration of tranexamic acid and reduced incidence of early rebleeding after aneurysmal subarachnoid hemorrhage: a prospective randomized study. J Neurosurg 2002;97(4):771–8.
15. Lowenstein DH, Alldredge BK. Status epilepticus at an urban public hospital in the 1980s. Neurology 1993;43(3 Pt 1):483–8.
16. Alldredge BK, Gelb AM, Isaacs SM, et al. A comparison of lorazepam, diazepam, and placebo for the treatment of out-of-hospital status epilepticus. N Engl J Med 2001;345(9):631–7.
17. Leys D, Ringelstein EB, Kaste M, et al, Executive Committee of the European Stroke Initiative. Facilities available in European hospitals treating stroke patients. Stroke 2007;38(11):2985–91.
18. Ganapathy K. Telemedicine and neurosciences. J Clin Neurosci 2005;12(8): 851–62.
19. Ragoschke-Schumm A, Walter S, Haass A, et al. Translation of the 'time is brain' concept into clinical practice: focus on prehospital stroke management. Int J Stroke 2014;9(3):333–40.
20. Shore JH. Telepsychiatry: videoconferencing in the delivery of psychiatric care. Am J Psychiatry 2013;170(3):256–62.
21. Wilcox ME, Adhikari NK. The effect of telemedicine in critically ill patients: systematic review and meta-analysis. Crit Care 2012;16(4):R127.
22. Levine SR, Gorman M. "Telestroke": the application of telemedicine for stroke. Stroke 1999;30(2):464–9.
23. Hess DC, Wang S, Hamilton W, et al. REACH: clinical feasibility of a rural telestroke network. Stroke 2005;36(9):2018–20.
24. Audebert HJ, Schwamm L. Telestroke: scientific results. Cerebrovasc Dis 2009; 27(Suppl 4):15–20.
25. Engelter ST, Gostynski M, Papa S, et al. Barriers to stroke thrombolysis in a geographically defined population. Cerebrovasc Dis 2007;23(2–3):211–5.
26. Silva GS, Schwamm LH. Use of telemedicine and other strategies to increase the number of patients that may be treated with intravenous thrombolysis. Curr Neurol Neurosci Rep 2012;12(1):10–6.
27. Hess DC, Audebert HJ. The history and future of telestroke. Nat Rev Neurol 2013;9(6):340–50.
28. Muller-Barna P, Schwamm LH, Haberl RL. Telestroke increases use of acute stroke therapy. Curr Opin Neurol 2012;25(1):5–10.
29. Agarwal S, Warburton EA. Teleneurology: is it really at a distance? J Neurol 2011;258(6):971–81.
30. Switzer JA, Demaerschalk BM. Overcoming challenges to sustain a telestroke network. J Stroke Cerebrovasc Dis 2012;21(7):535–40.
31. Diringer MN, Edwards DF. Admission to a neurologic/neurosurgical intensive care unit is associated with reduced mortality rate after intracerebral hemorrhage. Crit Care Med 2001;29(3):635–40.
32. Suarez JI, Zaidat OO, Suri MF, et al. Length of stay and mortality in neurocritically ill patients: impact of a specialized neurocritical care team. Crit Care Med 2004;32(11):2311–7.

33. Mirski MA, Chang CW, Cowan R. Impact of a neuroscience intensive care unit on neurosurgical patient outcomes and cost of care: evidence-based support for an intensivist-directed specialty ICU model of care. J Neurosurg Anesthesiol 2001;13(2):83–92.

34. Varelas PN, Conti MM, Spanaki MV, et al. The impact of a neurointensivist-led team on a semiclosed neurosciences intensive care unit. Crit Care Med 2004;32(11):2191–8.

35. Vespa PM, Miller C, Hu X, et al. Intensive care unit robotic telepresence facilitates rapid physician response to unstable patients and decreased cost in neurointensive care. Surg Neurol 2007;67(4):331–7.

36. Audebert HJ, Schultes K, Tietz V, et al. Long-term effects of specialized stroke care with telemedicine support in community hospitals on behalf of the Telemedical Project for Integrative Stroke Care (TEMPiS). Stroke 2009;40(3):902–8.

37. Shafqat S, Kvedar JC, Guanci MM, et al. Role for telemedicine in acute stroke. feasibility and reliability of remote administration of the NIH stroke scale. Stroke 1999;30(10):2141–5.

38. Wang S, Lee SB, Pardue C, et al. Remote evaluation of acute ischemic stroke: reliability of National Institutes of Health Stroke Scale via telestroke. Stroke 2003; 34(10):e188–91.

39. Handschu R, Littmann R, Reulbach U, et al. Telemedicine in emergency evaluation of acute stroke: interrater agreement in remote video examination with a novel multimedia system. Stroke 2003;34(12):2842–6.

40. Meyer BC, Raman R, Chacon MR, et al. Reliability of site-independent telemedicine when assessed by telemedicine-naive stroke practitioners. J Stroke Cerebrovasc Dis 2008;17(4):181–6.

41. Meyer BC, Lyden PD, Al-Khoury L, et al. Prospective reliability of the STRokE DOC wireless/site independent telemedicine system. Neurology 2005;64(6):1058–60.

42. Gonzalez MA, Hanna N, Rodrigo ME, et al. Reliability of prehospital real-time cellular video phone in assessing the simplified National Institutes of Health Stroke Scale in patients with acute stroke: a novel telemedicine technology. Stroke 2011;42(6):1522–7.

43. Anderson ER, Smith B, Ido M, et al. Remote assessment of stroke using the iPhone 4. J Stroke Cerebrovasc Dis 2013;22(4):340–4.

44. Demaerschalk BM, Vegunta S, Vargas BB, et al. Reliability of real-time video smartphone for assessing National Institutes of Health Stroke Scale scores in acute stroke patients. Stroke 2012;43(12):3271–7.

45. Craig JJ, McConville JP, Patterson VH, et al. Neurological examination is possible using telemedicine. J Telemed Telecare 1999;5(3):177–81.

46. Craig J, Russell C, Patterson V, et al. User satisfaction with realtime teleneurology. J Telemed Telecare 1999;5(4):237–41.

47. Chua R, Craig J, Wootton R, et al. Randomised controlled trial of telemedicine for new neurological outpatient referrals. J Neurol Neurosurg Psychiatr 2001; 71(1):63–6.

48. Johnston KC, Worrall BB, Teleradiology Assessment of Computerized Tomographs Online Reliability Study. Teleradiology Assessment of Computerized Tomographs Online Reliability Study (TRACTORS) for acute stroke evaluation. Telemed J E Health 2003;9(3):227–33.

49. Puetz V, Bodechtel U, Gerber JC, et al. Reliability of brain CT evaluation by stroke neurologists in telemedicine. Neurology 2013;80(4):332–8.

50. Schwamm LH, Rosenthal ES, Hirshberg A, et al. Virtual TeleStroke support for the emergency department evaluation of acute stroke. Acad Emerg Med 2004;11(11):1193–7.

51. Gross H, Hall C, Switzer JA, et al. Using tPA for acute stroke in a rural setting. Neurology 2007;68(22):1957–8 [author reply: 1958].

52. Audebert HJ, Schenkel J, Heuschmann PU, et al, Telemedic Pilot Project for Integrative Stroke Care Group. Effects of the implementation of a telemedical stroke network: the Telemedic Pilot Project for Integrative Stroke Care (TEMPiS) in Bavaria, Germany. Lancet Neurol 2006;5(9):742–8.

53. Sairanen T, Soinila S, Nikkanen M, et al. Two years of Finnish telestroke: thrombolysis at spokes equal to that at the hub. Neurology 2011;76(13):1145–52.

54. Rogove HJ, McArthur D, Demaerschalk BM, et al. Barriers to telemedicine: survey of current users in acute care units. Telemed J E Health 2012;18(1):48–53.

55. Switzer JA, Levine SR, Hess DC. Telestroke 10 years later–'telestroke 2.0'. Cerebrovasc Dis 2009;28(4):323–30.

56. LaMonte MP, Xiao Y, Hu PF, et al. Shortening time to stroke treatment using ambulance telemedicine: teleBAT. J Stroke Cerebrovasc Dis 2004;13(4):148–54.

57. Vespa PM. Multimodality monitoring and telemonitoring in neurocritical care: from microdialysis to robotic telepresence. Curr Opin Crit Care 2005;11(2): 133–8.

58. Rincon F, Vibbert M, Childs V, et al. Implementation of a model of robotic telepresence (RTP) in the neuro-ICU: effect on critical care nursing team satisfaction. Neurocrit Care 2012;17(1):97–101.

59. Brott T, Adams HP Jr, Olinger CP, et al. Measurements of acute cerebral infarction: a clinical examination scale. Stroke 1989;20(7):864–70.

60. Goldstein LB, Bertels C, Davis JN. Interrater reliability of the NIH stroke scale. Arch Neurol 1989;46(6):660–2.

61. Adams HP Jr, del Zoppo G, Alberts MJ, et al. Guidelines for the early management of adults with ischemic stroke: a guideline from the American Heart Association/American Stroke Association Stroke Council, Clinical Cardiology Council, Cardiovascular Radiology and Intervention Council, and the Atherosclerotic Peripheral Vascular Disease and Quality Of Care Outcomes in Research Interdisciplinary Working Groups: the American Academy of Neurology affirms the value of this guideline as an educational tool for neurologists. Stroke 2007; 38(5):1655–711.

62. Jauch EC, Saver JL, Adams HP Jr, et al. Guidelines for the early management of patients with acute ischemic stroke: a guideline for healthcare professionals from the American Heart Association/American Stroke Association. Stroke 2013;44(3):870–947.

63. Frank B, Fulton RL, Lees KR, VISTA Collaborators. The effect of time to treatment on outcome in very elderly thrombolysed stroke patients. Int J Stroke 2014;9(5): 591–6.

64. Lyerly MJ, Houston JT, Boehme AK, et al. Safety of intravenous tissue plasminogen activator administration with computed tomography evidence of prior infarction. J Stroke Cerebrovasc Dis 2014;23(6):1657–61.

65. Hacke W, Kaste M, Bluhmki E, et al. Thrombolysis with alteplase 3 to 4.5 hours after acute ischemic stroke. N Engl J Med 2008;359(13):1317–29.

66. Anile C, Zanghi F, Bracali A, et al. Sodium nitroprusside and intracranial pressure. Acta Neurochir (Wien) 1981;58(3–4):203–11.

67. Leigh R, Zaidat OO, Suri MF, et al. Predictors of hyperacute clinical worsening in ischemic stroke patients receiving thrombolytic therapy. Stroke 2004;35(8): 1903–7.

68. Illoh OC, Illoh K. Thrombolytic-associated coagulopathy and management dilemmas: a review of two cases. Blood Coagul Fibrinolysis 2008;19(6):605–7.

69. Khatri P, Wechsler LR, Broderick JP. Intracranial hemorrhage associated with revascularization therapies. Stroke 2007;38(2):431–40.
70. French KF, White J, Hoesch RE. Treatment of intracerebral hemorrhage with tranexamic acid after thrombolysis with tissue plasminogen activator. Neurocrit Care 2012;17(1):107–11.
71. Anderson CS, Heeley E, Huang Y, et al. Rapid blood-pressure lowering in patients with acute intracerebral hemorrhage. N Engl J Med 2013;368(25): 2355–65.
72. What you should know about cerebral aneurysms [Internet]: American Heart Association; 2014. Available at: http://www.strokeassociation.org/STROKEORG/AboutStroke/TypesofStroke/HemorrhagicBleeds/What-You-Should-Know-About-Cerebral-Aneurysms_UCM_310103_Article.jsp. Accessed July 10, 2014.
73. Sacco S, Marini C, Toni D, et al. Incidence and 10-year survival of intracerebral hemorrhage in a population-based registry. Stroke 2009;40(2):394–9.
74. Manno EM. Update on intracerebral hemorrhage. Continuum (Minneap Minn) 2012;18(3):598–610.
75. Fogelholm R, Murros K, Rissanen A, et al. Long term survival after primary intracerebral haemorrhage: a retrospective population based study. J Neurol Neurosurg Psychiatr 2005;76(11):1534–8.
76. Zumkeller M, Behrmann R, Heissler HE, et al. Computed tomographic criteria and survival rate for patients with acute subdural hematoma. Neurosurgery 1996;39(4):708–12 [discussion: 712–3].
77. Bederson JB, Connolly ES Jr, Batjer HH, et al. Guidelines for the management of aneurysmal subarachnoid hemorrhage: a statement for healthcare professionals from a special writing group of the Stroke Council, American Heart Association. Stroke 2009;40(3):994–1025.
78. van Asch CJ, Luitse MJ, Rinkel GJ, et al. Incidence, case fatality, and functional outcome of intracerebral haemorrhage over time, according to age, sex, and ethnic origin: a systematic review and meta-analysis. Lancet Neurol 2010;9(2):167–76.
79. Broderick JP, Brott TG, Duldner JE, et al. Volume of intracerebral hemorrhage. A powerful and easy-to-use predictor of 30-day mortality. Stroke 1993;24(7): 987–93.
80. Kowalski RG, Claassen J, Kreiter KT, et al. Initial misdiagnosis and outcome after subarachnoid hemorrhage. JAMA 2004;291(7):866–9.
81. Shea AM, Reed SD, Curtis LH, et al. Characteristics of nontraumatic subarachnoid hemorrhage in the United States in 2003. Neurosurgery 2007;61(6):1131–7 [discussion: 1137–8].
82. Wermer MJ, Kool H, Albrecht KW, et al, Aneurysm Screening after Treatment for Ruptured Aneurysms Study Group. Subarachnoid hemorrhage treated with clipping: long-term effects on employment, relationships, personality, and mood. Neurosurgery 2007;60(1):91–7 [discussion: 97–8].
83. Passier PE, Visser-Meily JM, Rinkel GJ, et al. Life satisfaction and return to work after aneurysmal subarachnoid hemorrhage. J Stroke Cerebrovasc Dis 2011; 20(4):324–9.
84. Suarez JI. Outcome in neurocritical care: advances in monitoring and treatment and effect of a specialized neurocritical care team. Crit Care Med 2006;34(9 Suppl):S232–8.
85. Frontera JA. Blood pressure in intracerebral hemorrhage–how low should we go? N Engl J Med 2013;368(25):2426–7.
86. Morgenstern LB, Hemphill JC 3rd, Anderson C, et al. Guidelines for the management of spontaneous intracerebral hemorrhage: a guideline for

healthcare professionals from the American Heart Association/American Stroke Association. Stroke 2010;41(9):2108–29.

87. Andrews CM, Jauch EC, Hemphill JC 3rd, et al. Emergency neurological life support: intracerebral hemorrhage. Neurocrit Care 2012;17(Suppl 1): S37–46.

88. Frontera JA. Decision making in neurocritical care. New York: Thieme Medical Publisher, Inc; 2009.

89. Connolly ES Jr, Rabinstein AA, Carhuapoma JR, et al. Guidelines for the management of aneurysmal subarachnoid hemorrhage: a guideline for healthcare professionals from the American Heart Association/American Stroke Association. Stroke 2012;43(6):1711–37.

90. Alberts MJ, Latchaw RE, Selman WR, et al. Recommendations for comprehensive stroke centers: a consensus statement from the brain attack coalition. Stroke 2005;36(7):1597–616.

91. Walter S, Kostopoulos P, Haass A, et al. Diagnosis and treatment of patients with stroke in a mobile stroke unit versus in hospital: a randomised controlled trial. Lancet Neurol 2012;11(5):397–404.

92. Ebinger M, Winter B, Wendt M, et al. Effect of the use of ambulance-based thrombolysis on time to thrombolysis in acute ischemic stroke: a randomized clinical trial. JAMA 2014;311(16):1622–31.

93. Audebert HJ, Kukla C, Vatankhah B, et al. Comparison of tissue plasminogen activator administration management between telestroke network hospitals and academic stroke centers: the Telemedical Pilot Project for Integrative Stroke Care in Bavaria/Germany. Stroke 2006;37(7):1822–7.

94. Schwab S, Vatankhah B, Kukla C, et al. Long-term outcome after thrombolysis in telemedical stroke care. Neurology 2007;69(9):898–903.

95. Hill MD, Buchan AM, Canadian Alteplase for Stroke Effectiveness Study (CASES) Investigators. Thrombolysis for acute ischemic stroke: results of the Canadian Alteplase for Stroke Effectiveness Study. CMAJ 2005;172(10): 1307–12.

96. Kohrmann M, Schellinger PD, Breuer L, et al. Avoiding in hospital delays and eliminating the three-hour effect in thrombolysis for stroke. Int J Stroke 2011; 6(6):493–7.

97. Schwamm LH, Starkman S. Have CT–will travel: to boldly go where no scan has gone before. Neurology 2013;80(2):130–1.

98. Gierhake D, Weber JE, Villringer K, et al. Technical aspects of prehospital stroke imaging before intravenous thrombolysis. Rofo 2013;185(1):55–9.

99. Weber JE, Ebinger M, Rozanski M, et al. Prehospital thrombolysis in acute stroke: results of the PHANTOM-S pilot study. Neurology 2013;80(2):163–8.

100. UTHealth introduces nation's first mobile stroke unit [Internet]. Houston (TX): UTHealth; 2014. Available at: https://www.uth.edu/media/story.htm?id=b1485cfc-110f-4a4c-91ea-06b573b3ba6d. Accessed July 14, 2010.

101. Meyer BC, Raman R, Hemmen T, et al. Efficacy of site-independent telemedicine in the STRokE DOC trial: a randomised, blinded, prospective study. Lancet Neurol 2008;7(9):787–95.

102. Demaerschalk BM, Bobrow BJ, Raman R, et al. Stroke team remote evaluation using a digital observation camera in Arizona: the initial Mayo Clinic experience trial. Stroke 2010;41(6):1251–8.

103. Demaerschalk BM, Bobrow BJ, Raman R, et al. CT interpretation in a telestroke network: agreement among a spoke radiologist, hub vascular neurologist, and hub neuroradiologist. Stroke 2012;43(11):3095–7.

104. Silbergleit R, Durkalski V, Lowenstein D, et al. Intramuscular versus intravenous therapy for prehospital status epilepticus. N Engl J Med 2012;366(7):591–600.
105. Brophy GM, Bell R, Claassen J, et al. Guidelines for the evaluation and management of status epilepticus. Neurocrit Care 2012;17(1):3–23.
106. Claassen J, Silbergleit R, Weingart SD, et al. Emergency neurological life support: status epilepticus. Neurocrit Care 2012;17(Suppl 1):S73–8.
107. Claassen J, Jette N, Chum F, et al. Electrographic seizures and periodic discharges after intracerebral hemorrhage. Neurology 2007;69(13):1356–65.

Outcomes Related to Telemedicine in the Intensive Care Unit
What We Know and Would Like to Know

Ramesh Venkataraman, MD, FCCM[a],
Nagarajan Ramakrishnan, MD, MMM, FCCM[b],*

KEYWORDS

- Telemedicine • Tele-ICU • Tele-monitoring • Tele-intensivist • Outcomes

KEY POINTS

- The Telemedicine Intensive Care Unit (Tele-ICU) seems to be well accepted by nurses and residents. However, its effect on physician job satisfaction and burnout and resident education is unknown.
- Tele-ICU enhances compliance with best care practices and care bundles and improves their sustenance.
- The impact of Tele-ICU on ICU/hospital length of stay and mortality is variable.
- Although Tele-ICU implementation incurs substantial costs, it may be cost-effective when the intensity of application is high and in sicker patients.
- Several crucial outcomes related to Tele-ICU remain unanswered.

INTRODUCTION

Telemedicine is defined as "the use of medical information exchanged from one site to another via electronic communications to improve patients' health status" (http://www.americantelemed.org/about-telemedicine/what-is-telemedicine#. Accessed January, 2015) and has been incorporated into various fields of medicine. Telemedicine now has been used in the intensive care setting for many decades. Although the employment of telemedicine technology to provide care in the intensive care unit (ICU) has been given several names (ie, Tele-ICU, virtual ICU, remote ICU, and eICU), they all refer to the provision of patient care by a centralized critical care

Disclosure: The authors have nothing to disclose.
This article has not been published previously in whole or part elsewhere.
[a] Department of Critical Care Medicine, Apollo Hospitals, 21 Greams Lane, Chennai 600 006, India; [b] Department of Critical Care Medicine, Apollo Hospitals, 21 Greams Lane, Chennai 600 006, India
* Corresponding author.
E-mail addresses: nramakrishnan@icumedicine.com; icudoctor@gmail.com

http://dx.doi.org/10.1016/j.ccc.2014.12.003
0749-0704/15/$ – see front matter © 2015 Elsevier Inc. All rights reserved.
criticalcare.theclinics.com

team (often based in a remote location) via constant 2-way interaction with the bedside ICU team and patients using audiovisual communication and computer systems. For the purposes of this review, the authors use the term *Tele-ICU* to describe the use of telemedicine to provide ICU care.

With the increasing use of Tele-ICU coverage, multiple investigators have evaluated the effect of Tele-ICU implementation on several relevant outcomes to understand its applicability, utility, impact, and cost-effectiveness. In a consensus statement on the research agenda in ICU telemedicine, the Critical Care Societies Collaborative[1] recommended that a comprehensive outcome evaluation should be done from the perspective of the provider, the patients, the health care system, and those responsible for paying for care. The authors have, hence, adapted this framework in this review to report the existing evidence and the lacunae relating to outcomes of Tele-ICU (**Fig. 1**).

TELEMEDICINE INTENSIVE CARE UNIT AND PROVIDER-CENTERED OUTCOMES

Tele-ICU provides for several important provider-centered outcomes. It can lessen the workload of the bedside intensivist and minimize the number of phone calls at off hours and, hence, enhance their quality of life and reduce burnout rates. Tele-ICU ensures easy access to an intensivist at all times of the day to the bedside nursing and technical staff and thereby gives them a sense of security and confidence to handle complex patient problems. This access is likely to have a positive influence on staff turnover and job satisfaction. Tele-ICU enables residents and fellows to discuss patient status, clinical decision making, and patient response with consultants in real time and obtain immediate feedback, which can augment their clinical experience and educational value. However, for Tele-ICU to have a positive impact on outcomes, it should be well accepted by the bedside clinical staff and must be easily adopted and integrated into a system without disrupting the workflow pattern.[1]

Staff Acceptance

Studies that have evaluated staff acceptance of Tele-ICU have provided variable results.[2-8] Many of these studies, however, are limited by a lack of rigorous methodology

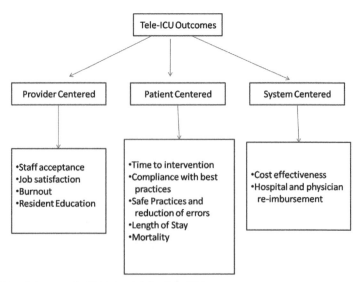

Fig. 1. An outcome evaluation model for Tele-ICU.

and use of survey instruments that were not validated. Shahpori and colleagues[2] evaluated the preimplementation knowledge and perceptions of ICU clinicians regarding the ability of Tele-ICU to address the human resource shortage and the provision of quality care. Using an online survey, the investigators found that before implementation there was overall low self-rated knowledge about Tele-ICU and significant uncertainty and skepticism among the intensivists regarding its ability to address human resource shortage and delivery of quality ICU care. However, a recent systematic review evaluated the acceptance of Tele-ICU coverage among ICU staff[3] and found that, despite initial ambivalence among nurses before implementation, the overall staff acceptance rate of Tele-ICU coverage was high, with a mean satisfaction score of 4.22 to 4.53 on a Likert scale of 1 to 5. In addition, 66.7% of residents training in ICUs equipped with Tele-ICU favored Tele-ICU support after their residency. Most of the study participants (>82%) also thought that Tele-ICU coverage favorably impacted patient outcomes. Similarly, most nurses surveyed in another study supported the use of Tele-ICU and, in addition, thought that personally knowing the Tele-intensivist was important (79%) and were more likely to contact the telemedicine unit if they knew the physician on duty (61%).[7] Tele-ICU training, understanding and expectations of the bedside staff, perceived need, and organizational factors, such as availability of resources for local coordination, have been identified as factors influencing the acceptance of Tele-ICU before its implementation.[8]

Job Satisfaction and Burnout

In a small case control model, Romig and colleagues[6] evaluated the impact of a nocturnal telemedicine service on nursing staff satisfaction and perceptions of quality of care. The investigators administered a modified version of a validated tool to ICU nurses before and 2 months after an experimental program of Tele-ICU. Nurses in another ICU within the same center where Tele-ICU was not implemented served as controls for the survey responses. Nurses exposed to Tele-ICU had a significant improvement in their survey scores after Tele-ICU implementation in specific subscales that addressed communication with other health workers, the psychological working conditions, burnout, and educational experience.

In another study, 50 nurses from 5 different Tele-ICUs were interviewed about their background, activities, work organization, sources of job satisfaction and dissatisfaction, and their motivation to work in the Tele-ICU.[9] This study reported that most Tele-ICU nurses were satisfied with their job; challenge in work and opportunity to learn were the most common motivation factors for these nurses to work in the Tele-ICU setting. Issues related to the working conditions, such as high mental workload, lack of physical activity, and layout of the Tele-ICU without windows, followed by missing clinical ICU work were the most frequently quoted factors for dissatisfaction. Unfortunately, no studies have evaluated the impact of implementation of a Tele-ICU program on the workload, quality of life, job satisfaction, and burnout rates of bedside intensivists, despite them being very important outcomes that could help alter the acceptance and application of this technology.

Resident Education

Tele-ICU has the potential to augment the educational experience of residents by enabling them to interact with consultants at all times and discuss complex patient problems and key management plans. However, the easy access to consultants round the clock could encourage the nursing and ancillary staff to call them directly with all patient management queries, thereby depriving trainees an opportunity to hone their communication and decision-making skills. A study evaluating resident perceptions of the impact of a Tele-ICU implementation on patient care, education, and the overall work environment[10] reported that most residents thought that this technology-based clinical support improved their ability to focus on urgent patient care issues and helped them to feel less overwhelmed. However, only 37% perceived Tele-ICU as a valuable educational experience. Many residents were also concerned about the impact of Tele-ICU on patient care continuity and communication. Despite these misgivings, Tele-ICU implementation was not perceived to have an overall negative impact on the educational experience.

Lacunae in Current Literature

Tele-ICUs have been a recent phenomena, and literature evaluating the perspectives of these caregivers is sparse. Caregivers at the Tele-ICU center are more likely to have reduced bedside clinical time and face-to-face interaction with patients and their families, work more night shifts, provide care without much continuity, and interact with staff at several ICUs with whom they may or may not have a professional rapport. These factors could adversely affect their job performance, satisfaction, and quality of life and increase their burnout rates. The optimal caregiver-to-patient ratio for remote monitoring has not been evaluated. Intuitively, too less a volume or too much of a patient load can contribute to professional dissatisfaction among the Tele-ICU staff. Future studies evaluating these critical outcomes could provide insight to improve the professional and personal wellbeing of the Tele-ICU professionals. The impact of Tele-ICU on the bedside clinical and procedural skills of caregivers also needs to be explored.

In summary (**Box 1**), existing literature in general points to the overall good bedside staff acceptance of Tele-ICU despite preimplementation skepticism and some concerns about privacy and its organizational impact. Factors that affect the acceptance and successful implementation of a Tele-ICU program need to be identified and targeted to provide optimal outcomes. There is paucity of data evaluating the optimal staffing model, job satisfaction, quality of life, and burnout rates among both the bedside and the Tele-ICU care team. Although most residents perceive Tele-ICU as a useful patient management resource, its impact on the educational experience is unclear.

TELEMEDICINE INTENSIVE CARE UNIT AND PATIENT-CENTERED OUTCOMES

The implementation of a Tele-ICU program in any given ICU intuitively improves patient care for several reasons. First, Tele-ICU extends intensivist coverage to ICUs that do not have an intensivist. Even in ICUs with an on-site intensivist, Tele-ICU will

---

Box 1
Provider-centered outcomes of Tele-ICU

- Tele-ICU is well accepted by nursing staff and residents.
- Education and training, clear delineation of bedside team responsibilities, and organizational support improve its acceptance.
- Bedside and Tele-ICU staff job satisfaction, quality of life, and burnout rates have not been evaluated.
- Optimal Tele-ICU staffing pattern is unknown.
- The influence of Tele-ICU on resident educational experience is unclear.

likely increase both the time during which an intensivist's input is available and the timeliness of an intensivist's input. Second, by virtue of continuous monitoring of patients using advanced alert systems, it enables caregivers to provide proactive rather than reactive care. Third, it provides for an extra layer of consultation and supervision at all times. Fourth, it can potentially increase adherence to best practices and care bundles. Finally, it influences the existing care process by increasing nurse and physician staffing and incorporating computerized order entry with checklists and smart alert systems for drug dosing and interactions and reducing medical errors. Although mortality is the primary patient-centered outcome and serves as the gold standard to ascertain the value of any intervention in the ICU, other equally important outcomes that need to be evaluated include patient safety, patient and family satisfaction, and health-related quality of life.[1] Although several studies have evaluated these outcomes in the context of Tele-ICU implementation, the existing literature is confounded by the lack of a standardized definition of Tele-ICU or how it is delivered or in what context it is delivered. Most studies have also been limited methodologically in that they are either retrospective, observational, or have used a preimplementation and postimplementation analysis.

Timeliness of Interventions

No major studies have compared the relative proportion of proactive and reactive patient care interventions or the response time to intervention for physiologic derangements in an ICU with and without Tele-ICU coverage. Only 6% of interventions were for prevention of physiologic instability in one survey.[11] A recent large multicenter observational study identified case review within 1 hour of ICU admission and quicker alert response times by the Tele-intensivist as individual components associated with improved outcomes.[12]

Compliance with Best Practices

Several studies have consistently documented that Tele-ICU implementation enhances compliance with various best practices in the ICU.[13–16] Youn[13] demonstrated that the Tele-ICU program enhanced compliance and documentation with 3 ventilator bundle components (ie, head-of-bed elevation, prophylaxis for deep venous thrombosis, and prophylaxis for stress ulcer prophylaxis). Although daily multidisciplinary rounds led by the Tele-intensivist alone had the least effect on ventilator bundle compliance, writing orders and then documenting the execution of these orders showed the greatest effect. Similarly, the addition of a night-shift Tele-ICU pharmacist increased the percentage of patients receiving a daily sedative interruption trial.[14] When the Tele-ICU team was given the authority to make all referrals to the organ procurement agency within the allotted time (1 hour of Glasgow Coma Scale <6 in ventilated patients), the rate of imminent death referrals increased drastically from 45% to 92%, with only one missed referral during the study period.[15] In a recent retrospective study, Kalb and colleagues[16] examined the effect of exposure to Tele-ICU–directed ventilator rounds on adherence to lung protective ventilation, ventilation duration ratio (VDR), and ICU mortality ratio. The investigators found that despite wide variability in adherence rates to low tidal volume ventilation before implementation across hospitals, there was a steady increase in the compliance rates with statistically significant improvement in the third quarter after implementation. More importantly, this improvement was sustained in the subsequent two-quarters. Similarly, VDR and ICU mortality ratio decreased significantly after the implementation of Tele-ICU–directed ventilator rounds.

Length of Stay and Mortality

The studies that have evaluated the effect of Tele-ICU service on key patient outcomes, such as length of ICU or hospital stay and mortality, have provided mixed results. In one of the first studies, evaluating outcomes related to Tele-ICU, Grundy and colleagues,[17] using a model of daily intensivist consultations via a 2-way audiovisual link between a small private hospital and a large university medical center, demonstrated that telemedicine was feasible, superior to telephone consultations, improved the educational experience, and influenced the process and quality of care in the critical care unit of the small hospital. In another study, management of ICU patients by an intensivists during a 16-week period using video conferencing and computer-based data transmission was shown to substantially decrease severity-adjusted ICU mortality, severity-adjusted hospital mortality, incidence of ICU complications, ICU length of stay (LOS), and ICU costs compared with 2 different 16-week periods within the year before the intervention during which time no on-site intensivist was available.[18] Although these two studies confirmed that Tele-ICU provision to smaller ICUs was feasible and improved quality of care and patient outcomes, they evaluated the use of Tele-ICU only in single, small ICUs with baseline low-intensity intensivist staffing.

To extend the value of this technology, the model should ideally allow tele-intensivists to care for patients in multiple ICUs and be able to favorably affect outcomes in the overall cohort of patients, even in ICUs with high intensity daytime intensivist staffing. Although large Tele-ICU service providers could attempt to cohort groups based on levels of services required, this may not always be feasible. Breslow and colleagues[19] examined the effect of a supplemental Tele-ICU care program, in 2 adult ICUs of a large tertiary care teaching hospital and demonstrated shorter ICU LOS and lower hospital mortality. The magnitude of the improvement was similar to those reported in studies examining the impact of implementing on-site dedicated intensivist staffing models. In a before-and-after study of more than 6000 patients conducted in a single academic center (7 different ICUs on 2 campuses), Tele-ICU intervention (compared with preintervention period) was associated with improvement in best practice adherence for the prevention of stress ulcers (96% vs 83%, respectively; odds ratio [OR] 4.57 [95% confidence interval (CI) 3.91–5.77]) and for the prevention of deep venous thrombosis prophylaxis (99% vs 85%, respectively; OR 15.4 [95% CI 11.3–21.1]); lower rates of preventable complications (1.6% vs 13.0% for ventilator-associated pneumonia [OR 0.15; 95% CI 0.09–0.23] and 0.6% vs 1.0%, respectively, for catheter-related bloodstream infection [OR 0.50; 95% CI 0.27–0.93]) reduced mortality (OR 0.42 [95% CI 0.31–0.52]) and decreased hospital LOS (9.8 vs 13.3 days, respectively; hazard ratio for discharge 1.44 [95% CI 1.33–1.56]).[20] There were significant improvements in care processes after the Tele-ICU implementation. The off-site intensivists performed a comprehensive review of all medical information available for new admissions, assessed patients using real-time video, and supplemented the admission plan when necessary. They also monitored patients continuously, responded to alarms, modified treatment plans as per patients' response, and communicated their input to the bedside team. This study identified a faster response to alerts for physiologic instability and care plan review of night admissions by the remote intensivist as elements of care associated with improved outcomes. The intense involvement of the Tele-ICU staff and the substantial changes to the care process likely had a positive effect on the study outcome. The effects of Tele-ICU interventions on crude and adjusted mortality and LOS were measured using a preassessment/postassessment model in a multicenter study involving 56 ICUs in 32 hospitals from 19 US health care systems.[12] The investigators reported significantly lower ICU and hospital LOS and mortality in the patients who received Tele-ICU coverage. Individual components of the interventions that were associated with improved outcomes were intensivist case review within 1 hour of admission, timely use of performance data, adherence to ICU best practices, and quicker alert response times. The biggest strength of this study was that it included several different types of ICUs and hospitals across many US regions making it broadly applicable.

Numerous studies have provided discordant results and have failed to show an outcome benefit with Tele-ICU coverage. A large systematic review and meta-analysis (13 studies, 27 hospitals, 35 ICUs, more than 41,000 patients) demonstrated that Tele-ICU coverage was associated with lower ICU mortality and LOS but not with lower in-hospital mortality or hospital LOS.[21] However, the ICUs included in this study differed significantly in their baseline staffing models and how the Tele-ICU was implemented or used, with almost half the ICUs included in the study using Tele-ICU only in the evenings and weekends. In addition, only some studies reported in-hospital mortality decreasing the statistical power to demonstrate a significant difference in this outcome. The investigators also found a lack of consistent measurement, reporting, and adjustment for patient severity among studies making it difficult to interpret the study results. The impact of Tele-ICU on outcomes was evaluated in a multicenter observational study (6 ICUs of 5 hospitals) in a large US health care system using a before-and-after study design.[22] The study found no significant differences in severity-adjusted ICU or hospital mortality or ICU or hospital LOS associated with the Tele-ICU intervention. However, the study demonstrated a significant interaction between the Tele-ICU intervention and severity of illness ($P<.001$) in which Tele-ICU was associated with improved survival in sicker patients. The negative results can be explained by the fact that the tele-intensivist staffing was available only from noon to 7 AM and the Tele-ICU team was delegated full treatment authority in only 31.1% of the patients. Similarly, another study of 4000 patients in 2 community hospitals did not find a reduction in ICU, non-ICU, or total mortality; hospital or ICU LOS; or hospital cost attributable to the introduction of Tele-ICU.[23] The study also revealed that neither continued presence nor the higher utilization of Tele-ICU improved the mortality. The outcomes of this study were confounded by the low baseline mortality of both ICU and non-ICU patients and the variable intensities of Tele-ICU coverage received by study patients, with only a minority of patients receiving high-level physician involvement. In a recent observational study, Nassar and colleagues[24] evaluated the impact of Tele-ICU on hospital LOS and ICU, hospital, and 30-day mortality within the US Department of Veterans Affairs health care system and found no outcome benefit with Tele-ICU monitoring and care. The study reported significant variability seen between ICUs in their readiness to adopt and implement Tele-ICU. This finding and the extremely low mortality rates of the control ICUs possibly resulted in the lack of outcome demonstration with Tele-ICU.

In essence, although various studies have provided conflicting results, certain patterns seem to clearly emerge (**Boxes 2** and **3**). When Tele-ICU is easily adopted and implemented, when it alters the care process substantially, and when Tele-ICU staff involvement is intense with full autonomy to decide, modify, and execute treatment plans, outcomes seem to be better.[12,19,20] Lilly and colleagues[12] reported that a major component of their intervention was the effort devoted to systems reengineering concurrent with the Tele-ICU implementation. This reengineering comprised the development and deployment of standardized protocols across all ICUs and induction of a strong culture of collaboration between bedside and Tele-ICU care teams. In contrast, in the studies that failed to show an outcome benefit, Tele-ICU was either not well accepted or used by bedside staff or applied with less intensity, both with regard to

---

Box 2
Patient-centered outcomes of Tele-ICU

- Tele-ICU improves compliance with best practices and care bundles.
- The effect on patient safety and medical errors is not studied.
- Family and patient satisfaction with Tele-ICU is not examined.
- The impact on ICU and hospital LOS and mortality is variable.

---

time and staff involvement.[23,24] In addition, the baseline mortality was also low in these studies indicating either low acuity of patients or a very high level of baseline care diluting the outcome benefits of Tele-ICU implementation. However, Tele-ICU was clearly associated with improved survival in sicker patients.[22]

Studies evaluating an intervention likely superior if not comparable with Tele-ICU, (ie, nighttime in-hospital intensivist staffing) have also not demonstrated outcome benefits.[25,26] Nighttime bedside intensivists may not add to the quality of care in ICUs with high-intensity daytime intensivist staffing[26] and when well-trained resident physicians with telephone access to intensivists provided off-hour patient care.[25] However, in ICUs with low-intensity daytime staffing, nighttime intensivist cover led to a decrease in severity-adjusted mortality.[26] Similarly, factors such as the intensity of daytime intensivist staffing, the acuity of patients admitted at off-hours, and the presence or absence of round-the-clock trained resident-physicians at the bedside may all affect the impact of Tele-ICU on patient outcomes.

Hence, studies evaluating the clinical outcomes of Tele-ICU should be interpreted with caution taking into account the nature of the actual intervention, the setting in which it is provided, the level of acceptance among bedside staff, the degree of compliance with Tele-ICU plans, the intensity of the intervention, and changes in care processes that accompany the Tele-ICU implementation.

TELEMEDICINE INTENSIVE CARE UNIT AND SYSTEM-CENTERED OUTCOMES

Key system-centered outcomes of Tele-ICU would include cost-effectiveness, physician and hospital reimbursement models, and its impact on work flow and referrals (**Box 4**).[1] The studies evaluating these outcomes are few and have provided mixed results.

Cost-effectiveness

One study evaluating the costs and effectiveness of a Tele-ICU program demonstrated a reduction in hospital and ICU mortality and 25% lower costs per case.[19]

Box 3
Factors that influence patient outcomes after Tele-ICU implementation

- Acceptance of the model by bedside staff
- Compliance of bedside staff with Tele-ICU recommendations
- Daytime intensity of intensivist staffing
- The level of Tele-ICU involvement in patient care
- The availability of quality nighttime bedside clinical staff
- Acuity and complexity of patients

Box 4
System-centered outcomes of Tele-ICU

- Capital and implementation costs are substantial.
- High-level Tele-ICU involvement in sicker patients seems to be cost-effective.
- Rigorous cost analysis is currently lacking.
- The impact of Tele-ICU on referrals out of or into an organization is unknown.
- No working model for tele-intensivist billing exists.
- The influence of Tele-ICU on bedside work flow is unclear.

This reduction in cost was attributable to a decrease in LOS leading to an increase in number of ICU cases per month by 7% and to lower daily ICU ancillary costs. However, another observational study of more than 4000 patients in 6 different ICUs found that the average daily costs (increase of 28%) and the costs per case increased in all the ICUs after implementation of the Tele-ICU.[27] There was a consistent increase of ICU costs across all ICUs and a clear increase in the Tele-ICU operational cost. The investigators reported that for patients with Simplified Acute Physiology Score (SAPS) II of 50 or less, Tele-ICU increased the cost of care without altering mortality. However, for a small proportion of patients (17%) with SAPS II greater than 50, Tele-ICU decreased mortality without significant increases in cost, making it cost-effective in this subset of sicker patients. The positive influence of Tele-ICU on ICU LOS and the cost-effectiveness in this study could have been annulled by the fact that Tele-ICU was delegated full responsibility for patient care only in a third of patients. These findings are concordant with another study that also demonstrated that the increase in hospital cost was steeper when there was only a low-level Tele-ICU involvement in patient care compared with when Tele-ICU involvement was high.[23] The largest systematic review evaluating the costs of Tele-ICU programs reported wide variability in the cost data published and estimated the cost of implementation and first-year operational cost of a Tele-ICU program to be between $50,000 and $100,000 per monitored ICU bed.[28] Tele-ICU implementation resulted in an in-hospital cost saving of $3000 to a $5600 cost increase per patient. The analysis of this study was limited in that several studies included in this review did not provide the costs for implementation, technology, or staffing. In addition, most studies did not report the cost per bed or cost per patient.

Studies evaluating the cost-effectiveness of Tele-ICU claim cost savings based on improvements in surrogate outcomes, such as LOS, ventilator days, and so forth. Future studies should provide the actual cost data in evaluating the cost-effectiveness of Tele-ICU. Several factors, such as cost incurred in the implementation of technology implementation, infrastructure necessary, and operational costs, including personnel and training costs, should be balanced against the cost of care and revenue generated from reimbursement.[29] Loss of revenue resulting from transferring outpatients and increased revenue from referrals resulting from enhanced capability to provide round-the-clock acute care must also be considered.

Currently, the cost-effectiveness of Tele-ICU implementation across all ICUs is unclear. High-level involvement by the Tele-ICU staff and management of sicker patients by the Tele-ICU seem to be cost-effective. The cost-effectiveness of Tele-ICU will vary depending on the structural and organizational characteristics of the institution, and individualized decisions need to made regarding the utility of Tele-ICU.

Hospital and Physician Reimbursement

Physicians and nurses providing Tele-ICU care are currently either employed by the organization on a salaried basis or paid on a per-shift basis. Currently, physicians are not able to directly bill patients for the Tele-ICU services they provide. A survey collected by the American College of Chest Physicians and the National Association for Medical Direction of Respiratory Care from 8 Tele-ICU programs in 2008 found that the average number of Tele-ICU encounters per site per 12-hour shift that could have been billed as critical care if they had been provided in person was only 1.75 (range, 0.16–2.62).[30] Many of the Tele-ICU interventions required less than 30 minutes, which is the minimum time needed for billing the encounter. Currently, the 2 Tele-ICU codes (*Current Procedural Terminology* [*CPT*] codes 0188T and 0189T) have been assigned to category 3 of *CPT*; hence, many payers do not recognize them for payment.[31] Moreover, some interventions that the tele-intensivist would bill for are likely considered to be part of the reimbursement of the bedside critical care physician; hence, it is unlikely that insurance providers would pay twice for the same service. But a recent survey of Tele-ICU interventions revealed that 80% of interventions were carried out when the bedside team was not available.[11] Therefore, reimbursement models that can be integrated within the existing system without affecting the revenue generated by the bedside intensivist service need to be explored. The inability of a Tele-ICU service to generate revenue along with the costs involved in establishment and sustenance of such a program seem to be a major reason for the recent slowing in the adoption of this technology.[32]

SUMMARY
What We Know

Given the increasing aging population and the severe shortage in intensivists,[33] innovative models to provide quality critical care need to be nurtured. The Tele-ICU model ideally serves this purpose and has been increasingly used to overcome this challenge created by supply/demand mismatch. Over the years, extensive research has been conducted evaluating various aspects of this technology.

Despite initial skepticism about its value, once implemented, Tele-ICU seems to be well accepted by nursing staff and residents.[2,3,10] Education of bedside staff about Tele-ICU, their roles and responsibilities, and the availability of organizational support seem to enhance acceptance. Residents in general like Tele-ICU and perceive it to be a good support system for patient management,[10] but its effect on their educational experience is unclear. Tele-ICU improves compliance with implementation and documentation of best practices and care bundles.[13–16] Giving full authority to the Tele-ICU team to implement these practices seems to sustain these practices.[16] Studies have provided conflicting results with regard to the influence of Tele-ICU on objective patient outcomes, such as ICU and hospital LOS and severity-adjusted mortality.[12,18–20,22–24] However, outcome benefits were consistently seen when Tele-ICU was easily adopted and integrated, when deployed in ICUs with low-intensity daytime intensivist staffing, when authorized for high-level involvement, and in sicker patients.[12,18–20] Like any other medical intervention, the context of application has to be carefully considered in interpreting these results. Although initial implementation costs can be substantial, Tele-ICU seems to be cost-effective in ICUs with low-intensity daytime staffing and when trained residents are not available to provide bedside care at nights. There is currently no working model for reimbursement for Tele-ICU services from insurance providers, and tele-intensivists are remunerated by the facility for their service.

What We Would Like to Know

Although the insight into various aspects of structure, function, and outcomes of Tele-ICU is increasing, several important issues still remain unanswered. The impact of Tele-ICU on bedside staff job satisfaction, quality of life, and burnout rates has not been studied. The optimal working conditions for the Tele-ICU team, like the nurse/patient ratio or physician/patient ratio, proportion of Tele-ICU shifts versus bedside shifts, and their job satisfaction, have not been elucidated. Studies need to evaluate whether predominant work in a Tele-ICU environment leads to attrition of clinical and procedural skills over time among nurses and physicians. Mechanisms to monitor and prevent this need to be investigated. The impact of Tele-ICU on resident education needs to be evaluated. and processes that can potentially augment it need to be implemented.

Despite the notion that Tele-ICU enables the provider to monitor patients continuously and provide proactive care, no major studies have reported the proportion of Tele-ICU interventions that prevent and treat physiologic instability or complications. The number of care plan interventions and modifications that require an intensivist-level input could indirectly assess the additive value of Tele-ICU. Because the tele-intensivist incorporates real-time video input of patients, monitors, and ventilator screens along with verbal reports from bedside staff, he or she is likely to make more accurate judgments of patient status, which could translate into better decision making. Whether this is actually true remains unanswered. Deployment of Tele-ICU could lead to ordering of more or less procedures, investigations, and imaging. The impact this has on the cost of care, patient safety, and outcomes has not been determined. Research is needed into the effect of Tele-ICU on medical errors, especially because bedside nursing staff could get disparate orders from the bedside and the tele-intensivist. Tele-ICU also has the potential to disrupt continuity of care, leading to redundancy in the care process and increasing resource utilization. The effect of Tele-ICU on patient and family satisfaction has not been examined in any major studies. The clinical impact of Tele-ICU will be related to the acceptance and subsequent execution of plans suggested by the Tele-ICU team. The current level of compliance with a Tele-ICU care plan and factors that could augment them have not been properly studied.

Most Tele-ICU outcome studies have used prestudy and poststudy design in which results could potentially be confounded by several covariables occurring in the system during the study period. Results have varied depending on the context of Tele-ICU implementation, type and intensity of intervention, and the collaborative culture in the study systems. Future studies should try standardizing these crucial variables and aim to prove causality of Tele-ICU implementation to outcomes rather than mere association. Other study designs, including cluster randomized trials or multicenter observational trials involving several health systems and Tele-ICU providers using ICUs without Tele-ICU coverage as controls, might provide more rigorous results.

The current literature is limited by the lack of transparent cost data and standardized methodology for cost-effectiveness assessment. The influence of Tele-ICU on referrals into or out of a health system remains unexplored. This influence could alter the revenue model impacting the cost-effectiveness. Robust cost-effective analysis should be undertaken based on the recommendations of the US Panel on Cost-Effectiveness in Health and Medicine.[34]

Institutions should independently weigh the costs and benefits of implementing and/or operating a Tele-ICU in the context of their health system before investing in this technology.

REFERENCES

1. Kahn JM, Hill NS, Lilly CM, et al. The research agenda in ICU telemedicine: a statement from the Critical Care Societies Collaborative. Chest 2011;140:230–8.
2. Shahpori R, Hebert M, Kushniruk A, et al. Telemedicine in the intensive care unit environment: a survey of the attitudes and perspectives of critical care clinicians. J Crit Care 2011;26:328.e9–15.
3. Young LB, Chan PS, Cram P. Staff acceptance of tele-ICU coverage: a systematic review. Chest 2011;139:279–88.
4. Chu-Weininger MY, Wueste L, Lucke JF, et al. The impact of a tele-ICU on provider attitudes about teamwork and safety climate. Qual Saf Health Care 2010;19:e39.
5. Berenson RA, Grossman JM, November EA. Does telemonitoring of patients: the eICU: improve intensive care? Health Aff (Millwood) 2009;28:w937–47.
6. Romig MC, Latif A, Gill RS, et al. Perceived benefit of a telemedicine consultative service in a highly staffed intensive care unit. J Crit Care 2012;27:426.e9–16.
7. Mullen-Fortino M, DiMartino J, Entrikin L, et al. Bedside nurses' perceptions of intensive care unit telemedicine. Am J Crit Care 2012;21:24–31.
8. Moeckli J, Cram P, Cunningham C, et al. Staff acceptance of a telemedicine intensive care unit program: a qualitative study. J Crit Care 2013;28:890–901.
9. Hoonakker PL, Carayon P, McGuire K, et al. Motivation and job satisfaction of Tele-ICU nurses. J Crit Care 2013;28:315–21.
10. Coletti C, Elliott DJ, Zubrow MT. Resident perceptions of a tele-intensive care unit implementation. Telemed J E Health 2010;16:894–7.
11. Lilly CM, Thomas EJ. Tele-ICU: experience to date. J Intensive Care Med 2010; 25:16–22.
12. Lilly CM, McLaughlin JM, Zhao H, et al. A multicenter study of ICU telemedicine reengineering of adult critical care. Chest 2014;145:500–7.
13. Youn BA. ICU process improvement: using telemedicine to enhance compliance and documentation for the ventilator bundle. Chest 2006;130(4_MeetingAbstracts): 226S–c.
14. Forni A, Skehan N, Hartman CA, et al. Evaluation of the impact of a tele-ICU pharmacist on the management of sedation in critically ill mechanically ventilated patients. Ann Pharmacother 2010;44:432–8.
15. Cowboy EN, Nygaard SD, Simmons R, et al. Compliance with CMS timely referral and organ procurement impact via Tele ICU. Chest 2009;136(4_MeetingAbstracts): 15S–b.
16. Kalb T, Raikhelkar J, Meyer S, et al. A multicenter population-based effectiveness study of teleintensive care unit-directed ventilator rounds demonstrating improved adherence to a protective lung strategy, decreased ventilator duration, and decreased intensive care unit mortality. J Crit Care 2014;29(4):691.e7–14.
17. Grundy BL, Crawford P, Jones PK, et al. Telemedicine in critical care: an experiment in health care delivery. JACEP 1977;6:439–44.
18. Rosenfeld BA, Dorman T, Breslow MJ, et al. Intensive care unit telemedicine: alternate paradigm for providing continuous intensivist care. Crit Care Med 2000;28:3925–31.
19. Breslow MJ, Rosenfeld BA, Doerfler M, et al. Effect of a multiple: site intensive care unit telemedicine program on clinical and economic outcomes: an alternative paradigm for intensivist staffing. Crit Care Med 2004;32:31–8.
20. Lilly CM, Cody S, Zhao H, et al. Hospital mortality, length of stay, and preventable complications among critically ill patients before and after tele-ICU reengineering of critical care processes. JAMA 2011;305:2175–83.

21. Young LB, Chan PS, Lu X, et al. Impact of telemedicine intensive care unit coverage on patient outcomes: a systematic review and meta-analysis. Arch Intern Med 2011;171:498–506.
22. Thomas EJ, Lucke JF, Wueste L, et al. Association of telemedicine for remote monitoring of intensive care patients with mortality, complications, and length of stay. JAMA 2009;302:2671–8.
23. Morrison JL, Cai Q, Davis N, et al. Clinical and economic outcomes of the electronic intensive care unit: results from two community hospitals. Crit Care Med 2010;38:2–8.
24. Nassar BS, Vaughan-Sarrazin MS, Jiang L, et al. Impact of an intensive care unit telemedicine program on patient outcomes in an integrated health care system. JAMA Intern Med 2014;174(7):1160–7.
25. Kerlin MP, Small DS, Cooney E, et al. A randomized trial of nighttime physician staffing in an intensive care unit. N Engl J Med 2013;368:2201–9.
26. Wallace DJ, Angus DC, Barnato AE, et al. Nighttime intensivist staffing and mortality among critically ill patients. N Engl J Med 2012;366:2093–101.
27. Franzini L, Sail KR, Thomas EJ, et al. Costs and cost-effectiveness of a telemedicine intensive care unit program in 6 intensive care units in a large health care system. J Crit Care 2011;26:329.e1–6.
28. Kumar G, Falk DM, Bonello RS, et al. The costs of critical care telemedicine programs: a systematic review and analysis. Chest 2013;143:19–29.
29. Kumar S, Merchant S, Reynolds R. Tele-ICU: efficacy and cost-effectiveness approach of remotely managing the critical care. Open Med Inform J 2013;7: 24–9.
30. McCambridge MM, Tracy JA, Sample GA. Point: should tele-ICU services be eligible for professional fee billing? Yes. Tele-ICUs and the triple aim. Chest 2011;140:847–9.
31. Hoffmann S. Counterpoint: should tele-ICU services be eligible for professional fee billing? No. Chest 2011;140:849–51.
32. Kahn JM, Cicero BD, Wallace DJ, et al. Adoption of ICU telemedicine in the United States. Crit Care Med 2014;42:362–8.
33. Angus DC, Kelley MA, Schmitz RJ, et al. Caring for the critically ill patient. Current and projected workforce requirements for care of the critically ill and patients with pulmonary disease: can we meet the requirements of an aging population? JAMA 2000;284:2762–70.
34. Understanding costs and cost-effectiveness in critical care: report from the second American Thoracic Society workshop on outcomes research. Am J Respir Crit Care Med 2002;165:540–50.

Telemedicine in the Intensive Care Unit

Its Role in Emergencies and Disaster Management

Daniel M. Rolston, MD, MS[a], Joseph S. Meltzer, MD[b],*

KEYWORDS

- Telemedicine • Tele-ICU • Tele-intensive care • Telemonitoring • Disaster
- Disaster response

KEY POINTS

- Earthquakes are the most deadly and the most costly of all natural disasters because of the large amount of damage to infrastructure that they inflict.
- Satellites are the most reliable method of communication and telemedicine after a disaster.
- Triaging patients to prioritize those who need the most urgent care is essential to disaster response and a potential area of improvement through telemedicine.
- Effective emergency mass critical care (EMCC) coordinates the use of medical equipment and supplies and hospital personnel and facilities to maximize survival of the greatest number of patients. Telemedicine has the ability to improve all areas of EMCC.
- Technological advances will improve smartphone and wireless monitoring in the future, which can greatly advance telemedicine in disasters and tele-intensive care units (ICUs).

INTRODUCTION

Telemedicine

The World Health Organization defines telemedicine as "The delivery of healthcare services, where distance is a critical factor, by all healthcare professionals using information and communication technologies for the exchange of valid information for diagnosis, treatment and prevention of disease and injuries, research and evaluation,

Disclosure statement: The authors have no disclosures to report. The authors do not accept any money or have any affiliations with outside organizations. No monetary funding was provided for writing this article.
[a] Department of Emergency Medicine, Ronald Reagan UCLA Medical Center, David Geffen School of Medicine at UCLA, 757 Westwood Plaza, Los Angeles, CA 90095, USA; [b] Department of Anesthesiology and Perioperative Medicine, Ronald Reagan UCLA Medical Center, David Geffen School of Medicine at UCLA, 757 Westwood Plaza, Suite 3325, Los Angeles, CA 90095-7403, USA
* Corresponding author.
E-mail address: jmeltzer@mednet.ucla.edu

Crit Care Clin 31 (2015) 239–255
http://dx.doi.org/10.1016/j.ccc.2014.12.004
0749-0704/15/$ – see front matter © 2015 Elsevier Inc. All rights reserved.

criticalcare.theclinics.com

and for continuing education of healthcare providers, all in the interests of advancing the health of individuals and their communities."[1] Telemedicine has evolved from the transmission of information via telephone in the early 1900s to video transmission by microwave in the 1960s to telesurgery via satellite transmission in the 2010s.[2]

Telemedicine can be delivered either in real time or as store-and-forward information. Real-time telemedicine provides the benefits of interaction, examination, data collection, and monitoring; however, it often requires high bandwidth (data transfer rate) especially if videoconferencing is being used. Store-and-forward telemedicine is typically used for electrocardiography (ECG), radiology, or photographs. It requires less bandwidth and can be accomplished with less reliable networks.[2]

Tele-ICU

With the unequal distribution of intensivists in the United States, tele-intensive care or tele-ICUs have been proposed and have been used as a way to fulfill the shortages. Several studies and a meta-analysis have found a benefit to implementation of a tele-ICU[3–5]; however, others have not,[6] including a before-and-after study from the Veterans Affairs Hospitals, which found no improvement in mortality or length of stay with the addition of a tele-ICU program.[7] Tele-ICUs are generally organized in a centralized or decentralized model. In the centralized model, the telemedicine center is a specific location with physicians and nurses who typically provide care 24 hours a day to many different hospitals. A centralized model has and can continue to be implemented in disasters because an incident command center, while functioning to organize the response to a disaster, could also provide a centralized location for consultation to local hospitals, overflow facilities, or mobile ICUs. Although the centralized model provides an organized approach to telemedicine with more stable means of communication, this model is likely to be more expensive because it requires overhead, consisting of a permanent to semipermanent location equipped with technology to provide intensive care response.

Large disasters would likely involve a combination of a centralized and a decentralized model. The decentralized model is organized with the ICU or mobile ICU at the center, and then telemedicine consultation is provided from multiple individual locations.[2] This model can be used for nighttime rounding by a staff of intensivists, who all have access to a telemedicine workstation at home. It has been used in the disaster setting, during a blizzard in the Baltimore area in 2010; however, this was a situation in which the decentralized model with a robot for nighttime rounding was already in place before the disaster.[8] The decentralized model may also be useful to obtain specialist consultation, such as a dermatologist or infectious disease physician to evaluate a rash seen in many survivors of a hurricane. As the smartphone technology improves, this model will likely become easier to use and less expensive because the telemedicine consultant will not need to be at a telemedicine workstation. Telemedicine "apps" have already been created and could be ideal in the disaster setting. In addition, tele-ICUs can also be organized in continuous care, scheduled care, reactive care, or consultative care models. Scheduled care is typically used for nighttime rounds, whereas reactive care involves an on-call telemedicine consult. Consultative care refers to the use of telemedicine for consultation on cases when additional expertise is needed.[2]

DISASTERS

The Centre for Research on the Epidemiology of Disasters (CRED) defines disaster as "a situation or event, which overwhelms local capacity, necessitating a request to national or international level for external assistance."[9] In addition, for a disaster to be entered into their database, they must fulfill one or more of the following criteria: (1) at least 10 people were killed, (2) at least 100 people were injured, (3) declaration of a state of emergency, or (4) call for international assistance. CRED maintains EM-DAT, the International Disaster Database, which allows open access searching at www.emdat.be. CRED is based at the School of Public Health of the Catholic University of Louvain in Belgium Disasters and receives international funding. Internationally, damages from natural disasters were in excess of US$ 118 billion, in 2013, the fifth lowest since 2003.

In general, disasters are classified as natural or man-made and are then subdivided by classification. Natural disasters have been further categorized by CRED: Geophysical (earthquake, volcano, avalanche); Meteorologic (storm, tornado); Hydrological (flood); Climatological (extreme temperature, drought, wildfire); Biological (infectious disease epidemic, insect infestation, animal stampede). Earthquakes are the most costly and deadly of all natural disasters. In the past 30 years, earthquakes were responsible for 29% of natural disaster deaths. However, the burden of deaths from earthquakes has increased in recent years, accounting for 58% of natural disaster deaths from 2000 to 2009.[10] These data do not include the earthquake in Haiti on January 12, 2010, that claimed the lives of more than 225,000 people. The reason for the increase in mortality may be because more than half of the 130 largest cities worldwide are located in earthquake-prone areas.[2] As the population expands and urbanization increases, the fatality rates from earthquakes and other natural disasters will continue to grow if the stability of buildings and other structures is not improved.[11] The costs from all natural disasters are also extraordinarily high. Internationally, economic losses from natural disasters were $118.6 billion in 2013 but averaged $156.7 billion from 2003 to 2012.[9] In the United States, the National Oceanic and Atmospheric Administration's National Climatic Data Center reports that natural disasters cost the United States $110 billion in 2012 and $23 billion in 2013.[12]

Man-made disasters range from chemical and radiation releases like the Chernobyl nuclear plant accident to terrorism and acts of war. Terrorism is designed to be both shocking and unpredictable, and it causes a large number of casualties internationally. According to the US State Department's National Consortium for the Study of Terrorism and Responses to Terrorism, 17,891 people died and 32,577 were wounded as a result of international terrorism in 2013.[13] The costs in response to terrorism can also be extraordinarily high. Ten years after the September 11,2011, terrorist attacks, the New York Times estimated that the overall cost to the United States was approximately $3.3 trillion, when including losses and the response of the "War on Terror."[14] Approximately $55 billion of this cost estimate is attributed to infrastructure damage, loss of life, injury, and cleanup. Telemedicine and tele-ICU have the potential to improve triage and early management of critically ill patients in the overwhelmed health care setting that occurs after a terrorist attack.

WARS AND THE MILITARY APPROACH

Wars are different from most other disasters because their timing is more predictable and militaries have more resources to prepare for the anticipated medical consequences of war. However, the casualties, dehydration, starvation, and loss of shelter during war are massive, posing major challenges for providing health care. Wars are classified by the United Nations as a "humanitarian crisis in a country, region or society where there is total or considerable breakdown of authority resulting from internal or external conflict and which requires an international response that goes beyond the mandate or capacity of any single agency and/or ongoing United Nations country program."[1] Telemedicine has been used during wars especially the most recent Afghanistan and Iraq wars; however, there is also potential for telemedicine to be used in the recovery of war-torn areas. Long after wars end, the after effects of war can cause long-standing consequences to the population. For example, the presence of land mines ravage war-torn areas for years to come and multiple international efforts are ongoing to try to eliminate the burden of land mines in these areas. Militaries have valued the scope that telemedicine has to offer, and they currently organize the most sophisticated telemedicine programs in the world. As a result, most of the advances in telemedicine seen today are developed by the military. One of the most important parts of military medicine is procedural and organizational standardization, which includes creating common terminology. Common terminology is important to improve communication between teams. Because of these advances in communication and organization, the North Atlantic Treaty Organization now aims to share resources and coordinate with multinational organizations to improve medical care.[2]

MEDICAL CONSEQUENCES FOLLOWING A DISASTER

The most common primary injuries sustained from a disaster are secondary to trauma from structural damage; however, asphyxia from dust inhalation, hypothermia and hyperthermia, burns, and electrical injuries are all possibilities after large structural damage.[15] Although the initial event is devastating, most deaths may not occur immediately. It is estimated that approximately 80% of deaths occur in the 3 days following an earthquake.[2,11] Secondary illnesses can occur from exposure to contaminated air or water, psychiatric problems like depression or posttraumatic stress disorder, or loss of access to care. Analysis of Hurricane Katrina and Hurricane Sandy data identified that a large proportion of morbidity and mortality occurred in the weeks after the disaster as patients with chronic medical illnesses lost access to care. Patients on dialysis lost access to their dialysis centers; patients ran out of their medications and supplies, which could not be refilled because of pharmacy closures; the elderly and chronically ill became trapped because of poor mobility and loss of power.[16–18] Closure of hospitals as a result of damage to the health care infrastructure can also be detrimental. Following Hurricane Sandy in New York, 6300 patients were evacuated to neighboring hospitals. Even in the months after Hurricane Sandy, there was a 20% increase in the number of patients cared for at the unaffected hospitals.[10] With such a large proportion of sick patients requiring prolonged care after disasters, additional support is likely to be beneficial. Telemedicine may provide additional physicians and nurses to support the overburdened health care systems after a disaster.

Terrorist attacks seem to follow a different injury pattern because most patient mortality occurs immediately as patients die as a result of their initial injuries. Although the health care system is overwhelmed, most patients transferred to the hospital immediately following prior terrorist attacks are not critically ill. Nine hundred eleven patients were received by two affiliated hospitals from the World Trade Center attack. Seven hundred seventy six patients (85%) were walking wounded, sustaining mild inhalation and eye irritant injuries. One hundred thirty five (15%) were admitted with 18 (13%) of these undergoing surgery. Twenty two of the 23 transfers were from the community hospital to specialized orthopedic or burn centers. Of the 109 patients admitted to Hospital A, 30 were to the surgical service. The mean ISS score of these patients was 12. There were 4 deaths (within minutes of arrival at the hospital) and 6 delayed deaths (day 1-14). Excluding walking wounded and DOAs, the critical mortality rate was 37.5% overall.[19] In addition, following the Madrid train explosions on March 11, 2004, 9% of those injured died immediately, whereas 12% of patients treated at the nearest hospital were in critical condition and 17% of these critically ill patients died.[20] Finally, following the London bombings on July 7, 2005, 7% of patients died immediately, whereas 3% of patients triaged on the scene were critically ill, of which 15% died.[21] Although most patients are not critically ill, terrorist attacks still lead to a large increase in the number of patients requiring treatment in an ICU.

DISASTER MANAGEMENT AND THE ROLE OF TELEMEDICINE
Planning and Preparedness

As the military has shown, the most important aspect of managing the health care crisis that occurs after a disaster is developing a plan to prepare for disaster response. Planning begins with risk assessment and risk avoidance measures to limit the effects of anticipated disasters, otherwise known as mitigation,[2] which may include anything from designing and constructing buildings that are resistant to earthquakes to antiterrorism intelligence efforts. A large portion of planning involves preparing to respond to a disaster, which includes the organizational response, acquisition of resources, and development of a disaster warning system. Because many health care providers are not involved in multiple disasters, the best way to prepare for disasters is with simulated exercises. Disaster education for the health care system with simulated exercises helps providers, hospitals, and organizations evaluate their ability to respond and flaws in the system. For telemedicine to be an effective part of the response, simulations on how to use telemedicine technologies are essential for responders to learn the often-unfamiliar technology.[12,22]

The incident command system is used by many emergency management organizations and provides a chain of commands for emergency response. Telemedicine is still not widely integrated into disaster management organizations and infrastructure but could be used to coordinate multiple aspects of response. Designating a telemedicine leader within the incident command system could improve planning, communication, and coordination of disaster relief efforts. In large, unanticipated disasters, assistance from multiple different organizations such as the World Health Organization, Red Cross, and militaries is essential to limiting the medical catastrophe.[2] Because these organizations do not have the same disaster response system, telemedicine could be used to maximize the efficiency of the overall response. For example, following the earthquake in Haiti, multiple humanitarian organizations responded; however, they had difficulty communicating with each other because of poor telecommunication technology and coordination.[23]

Utilities and Devices

For any telemedicine program to function reliably, power must be consistent throughout the disaster response. However, disasters frequently disrupt the electric grid, leading to power outages or unstable power conditions. A secondary power source is crucial to increase connectivity after a disaster. Gasoline or diesel generators are commonly used; however, solar or wind-powered generators are becoming more common, as are fuel cells. Ideally, the backup system would automatically begin functioning when the electric grid fails to preserve backup resources.[2]

Computer platforms, phones, servers, digital cameras, and network devices must all be available after a disaster to provide telemedicine. This requirement presents a potential problem for implementation of telemedicine if the right technology is not available. Video teleconferencing (VTC) systems are essential to providing real-time telemedicine in a disaster. In addition to video, physiologic monitors, radiology images, and laboratory data can be displayed on the screen with VTC. A hard end point refers to a VTC system or other device designed for telemedicine, whereas a soft end point refers to a personal computer or smartphone to provide audio, video, and data. Soft end points are becoming increasingly capable of telemedicine as technology advances. One branch of telemedicine is referred to as mobile health, which uses smartphones to provide health care consultation through their associated health care applications. To transmit this large quantity of data over long distances, a coder-decoder is used to compress the data.[2] The rapid improvements in technology will continue improve the delivery of telemedicine in the future.

Telemedicine Connectivity

Using telemedicine after a disaster can be difficult because participants need to be able to communicate continuously through data transfer, video conferencing, voice communication, or e-mail. Because disasters disrupt or overwhelm standard communication systems, a portable mode of connectivity and Internet connection is important. For these reasons, amateur radio and satellite systems are the most reliable, but there are some more common technologies that can also be used. Bluetooth technology can be used in the short range to connect computers and portable medical devices to a central workstation. Wireless local area networks, such as Wi-Fi networking, allow multiple different workstations to connect wirelessly and can be crucial for coordinating medical care in the area of a disaster. The major downside is the need for a preexisting Internet connection, which is often disrupted during a disaster. Mobile broadband is another possible source of Internet connection. It uses smartphones and cellular data networks to create a wireless network and connect with other devices; however, cellular data networks can be easily damaged and quickly overwhelmed during a disaster. The global system for mobile communications (3G, 4G) continues to expand, and the speed of mobile broadband will continue to increase dramatically as cellular providers invest more money.[2,24] Therefore, mobile broadband may become increasingly useful during disasters as the ability to overburden the system decreases with time.

Following a disaster, satellites likely provide the most reliable and expansive form of connectivity. Infrastructure, cell towers, and power may be lost, leaving satellite as the only reliable means of communication. However, satellites need to transmit data over large distances, so one of their problems is a high latency time, which makes video conferencing difficult. Satellites of differing altitudes can be used, varying from geosynchronous to low earth orbit. The larger the distance between satellites, the higher the latency time. In addition, the bandwidth (the speed of data transfer) of satellites used to be much lower than digital subscriber lines or cable, but recent advances in technology and the generation of broadband global area networks have improved the available bandwidth. However, these systems can still be expensive. Very small aperture terminal (VSAT) is another form of satellite that was designed to transmit small bits of data back to other terminals or hubs. They can transmit these data real time and are easily portable, making them ideal for responders out in the field during a disaster. The cost of satellite technology can be substantial, but another benefit of VSAT technology is that it is more affordable than broadband global area networks and the bandwidth is increasing as technology improves.[2,15]

T carrier lines are high-speed digital network transport services that provide low latency times and high bandwidth, allowing for videoconferencing, telesurgery, extensive downloading and uploading, and real-time communication. However, T carrier lines are expensive to set up and maintain, must be in place before a disaster, and can be disrupted by damage to infrastructure. However, T carrier lines can still be useful in the tele-ICU setting. Because critically ill patients require such extensive monitoring, the best place to take care of these patients is typically in hospitals that were not damaged by the disaster. If patients are able to be evacuated to a nearby hospital with T carrier lines in place that connect to another hospital, telemedicine center, or the Internet in general, tele-ICU becomes much easier.[2]

An example of the challenges of access to telecommunication technologies was seen following the Great East Japan Earthquake on March 11, 2011. Satellite mobile phones functioned correctly in 10 of the 14 disaster base hospitals. In addition, multichannel wireless access systems were installed at 13 of the disaster base hospitals and an additional 12 emergency hospitals. On day 0, these wireless access systems worked 72% of the time, but by day 1 to 3, they only worked 64% of the time, largely because of infrastructure damage. In the severely damaged areas, fixed-line phones, the Personal Handy-phone System, and the Internet did not work in the first 4 days, but some mobile phones worked by day 2. These ordinary means of communication functioned in less than 40% of the hospitals in the mildly damaged areas and seem to be an unreliable means of communication planning for a disaster.[25] Further evidence that one should not rely on standard telecommunication technologies comes from the earthquake in Haiti in 2010, where cell phone service was not restored for at least 17 days in Port-au-Prince.[20] Again, satellites seem to be the most reliable communication for large disasters; however, mobile phone technology is improving rapidly.

Triage

Many triage systems evaluate patients in the prehospital setting and coordinate care between the emergency department (ED) and ICU; however, during disasters, resources become limited and all aspects of patient care within the health system must be considered. To ensure that the population affected by a disaster is given the best chance of survival, disaster management officials must coordinate the utilization of scarce resources. The Center for Public Health Preparedness and Disaster Response recommends a multitiered approach: (1) At the community level, information must be provided on how to decrease risk exposure and spread of disease while also providing information on how to recognize illness and access care and shelter; (2) In the prehospital setting, patients should be appropriately distributed throughout the health care system, with the use of valid field triage protocols to ensure that only the patients who require the most urgent care are sent to hospitals; (3) On arrival at the hospital, patients should be rapidly stabilized until definitive care can be established, and the hospital should be organized to operate as efficiently as possible; (4) At the regional level, health emergency operations centers (HEOCs) must continually reassess the needs and allocation of resources.[26] Telemedicine can be especially useful for the HEOCs to communicate and evaluate the needs at each level to ensure that all aspects of the health care system are functioning as effectively and efficiently as possible.

Patient Triage

During disasters, early access to patients can be difficult. Because most disasters are unpredictable and international support typically takes 48 to 72 hours to arrive, the initial response requires local people and resources to support the relief efforts.[2,27] Immediately after a disaster, assistance with coordination of patient triage and medical logistics can be crucial to improved patient survival, so telemedicine could be helpful to visually triage patients or teach local, inexperienced responders how to appropriately triage patients. Effectively managing prehospital care can decrease the burden on first responders and hospital-based health care providers. Because medical resources are scarce during a disaster, avoiding unnecessary emergency transport becomes important. Patients with non–life-threatening illnesses can quickly overwhelm a small temporary field medical facility or a hospital if patients are inappropriately transported; therefore, an appropriate triage protocol is crucial to the initial response. Several primary mass-casualty triage protocols are available to identify patients in need of urgent treatment. In general, the protocols classify patients similarly (with color tags) based on the urgency of treatment: (1) deceased or expectant (black), (2) immediate (red), (3) delayed (yellow), or (4) ambulatory (green). The Simple Treatment and Rapid Transport (START) algorithm is used by many emergency medical services (EMS) systems in the United States, whereas the Care Flight Triage algorithm is used by many EMS systems in Australia. Both use an assessment of ability to walk, breathing, presence of pulse, and mental status in their algorithm.[28] There is some research on which algorithm is most effective; however, one does not seem to be better than the other. START and Care Flight Triage were found to have similar sensitivity; however, Care Flight Triage had higher specificity in the adult and pediatric population.[29,30] Because disasters often require international assistance, creating an international mass-casualty triage protocol would likely lead to a more efficient medical response to a disaster; however, more research seems necessary before a consensus can be made. In addition, telemedicine can be used to teach large groups of volunteers triage algorithms in a disaster, so consideration should be made for establishing a triage protocol that is easy to teach inexperienced providers.

Decreasing the burden on health care providers in the aftermath of a disaster is a critical part of any emergency response. A retrospective chart review revealed that 15% of patients transported to the hospital by ambulance could be managed by an EMS provider through telemedicine consultation with an emergency physician.[31] In addition, video telemedicine has been found to decrease the need for aeromedical evacuation of patients by 14% when compared with traditional telephone conversations[32] and by 36.2% when combined with screening criteria and a transfer protocol.[33] Decreasing aeromedical transport is particularly important during a disaster because of the loss of transportation infrastructure. Telemedicine can also be used to ensure that patients are triaged to the correct setting and the medical team is prepared to care for them. For example, transmitting ECGs to an attending cardiologist's mobile phone decreased the door-to-percutaneous coronary intervention (PCI) time by 63 minutes for patients with ST-segment elevation myocardial infarction. These patients were referred directly to a PCI center, where they could quickly receive appropriate care; this only increased the 911-to-door time by 8 minutes without any increased adverse events.[34]

Because the medical infrastructure is so dismantled during a disaster, many of the first responders have inadequate medical training to care for the severity of illness they encounter. Telemedicine can play a significant role in caring for the sick and injured by allowing paramedics, nurses, and physicians to visualize patients and communicate with surrogate caregivers in the field. There is minimal research on the use of telemedicine in inexperienced caregivers; however, first responders and providers referring for telemedicine-assisted care have increased confidence in their management and decision making.[14,35,36]

Some disasters, especially infectious disease outbreaks or bioterrorism, require quarantining patients and requesting that other patients remained sheltered in place. As long as the Internet is still available, Web-based systems could be used to provide patient consultation without putting others at risk. This same system could be used at nursing homes, workplaces, or any other location where an attack or outbreak may be suspected.[2] Following the sarin attacks in the Tokyo subway in 1995, secondary exposure to sarin caused 9.9% of the emergency medical technicians to develop acute sarin poisoning symptoms.[37] Most exposures were attributed to poor ventilation in the ambulance during transport of patients to the hospital, which improved once it was noticed by the control center. A vertically structured EMS system was in place in Tokyo, and poor communication between organizations was noted as one of the major problems with their disaster response.[37] Improved communication with telemedicine may have improved the overall response, especially with regards to secondary exposure.

In bioterrorism, video triage of patients could also help to limit the secondary exposure of emergency providers and identify the need for early decontamination of patients. Robots with videoconferencing capabilities could be sent into inhospitable climates or areas involved in bioterrorism to assist in triage and prepare providers for the potential chemical exposures. Robots have been used in a pediatric disaster simulation for specialist physician consultation with apparent success.[38] As previously mentioned, a robot was used to successfully provide medical consultation during the Baltimore blizzard of 2010[8]; however, the authors were unable to find any reports of robots being used for telemedicine in inhospitable climates or bioterrorism disasters. A HazBot robot was developed specifically for bioevent disaster response, but there are no reports of its use in a disaster.[39]

Resource Triage

Resource triage coordinates the allocation of health care resources to improve survival of the largest number of patients possible. Because there are ethical controversies and societal ramifications, this is usually done in coordination with regional and federal public health authorities.[31] Telemedicine is essential for the coordination of resource triage during a disaster, which most likely occurs at HEOCs or Incident Command Centers, and these centers may be long distances from the disaster. The Sequential Organ Failure Assessment (SOFA) score provides an objective measure of short-term survival of critically ill patients,[40] so it has been proposed as a useful tool to allocate resources for critically ill patients during a disaster.[41] White and colleagues[42] also proposed a multiprinciple allocation strategy that incorporates the prognoses for short-term (SOFA score) and long-term survival (based on medical comorbidities) while giving priority to younger patients because ethically they have had less chance to live through life's stages. Again, telemedicine can become extremely useful by providing consultation and multiple opinions in the situation when resources become scarce and a physician believes he/she should remove one patient from a life-sustaining treatment to treat another patient. There may be legal ramifications in this potential scenario, so additional medical opinions would become beneficial.

Tele-ICU

Because disasters are so unpredictable, they can quickly exhaust ICUs. Although the ED may be overwhelmed for hours to days after a disaster, patients admitted to the ICU can require weeks to even months of treatment. Following the London bombings in 2005, the triage of patients in the ED took 3 hours 14 minutes, while the average duration of stay of patients admitted to the ICU was 12.4 days. Additional help will likely be needed, and one possible avenue of assistance is through tele-ICU coverage.

EMCC uses a multimodality approach to resource utilization to maximize the number of survivors who can receive sufficient critical care (**Table 1**).[43,44] Medical equipment and supplies can become deficient quickly during a disaster. In the event of a disaster causing many patients to experience respiratory failure, such as a flu pandemic or large fire, ventilators and oxygen become limited resources, which must only be dispersed when absolutely necessary. A shortage of hospital personnel

Table 1
Emergency mass critical care and the potential for telemedicine

Phase of EMCC	Needs/Deficiencies	Potential for Telemedicine
Medical equipment and supplies	Ventilators, oxygen, dialysis, monitors, electricity	Recognize deficiencies; coordinate delivery of supplies; incident command center monitoring
Hospital personnel	Physicians, radiologists, nurses, respiratory therapists, dialysis nurses; sleep; stress relief	Tele-ICU; telemonitoring; teleradiology; telesurgery; telemedicine triage; specialist consultation; staff communication with family
Facilities	ICU beds, operating rooms, monitored beds	Coordinate bed control; wireless monitoring; incident command center monitoring; telemedicine triage

Data from Burke RV, Berg BM, Vee P, et al. Using robotic telecommunications to triage pediatric disaster victims. J Pediatr Surg 2012;47(1):221–24.

is often another issue. Even if there are enough intensive care physicians on staff, the damage to transportation infrastructure may make it impossible for staff to reach the hospital. As discussed previously, a case report out of Baltimore during 3 blizzards in the winter of 2009–2010 revealed that having a previously decentralized tele-ICU in place allowed intensive care physicians to round with nurses and house officers from home for 24 hours without untoward events.[8] A decentralized tele-ICU would be difficult to establish during a disaster, but it likely works well in a preestablished model. Protection of hospital staff from illness is paramount during bioterrorism and infectious disease outbreaks. Early identification, decontamination, and personal protective equipment including negative pressure respirators (N95 mask) are critical to prevent injury to staff. Another possible way to decrease exposure is by using telemedicine to visualize, triage, and treat patients. According to the American College of Chest Physicians guidelines, hospitals should be equipped to deliver EMCC for 10 days following a disaster.[45] Therefore, critical care physicians could be working very long hours in an extremely strenuous environment for a prolonged period. Telemedicine could alleviate some of the patient load or provide monitoring of critically ill patients while the physician sleeps. Space for patients is the third modality in the EMCC approach. Critical care requires highly complex technical equipment, electricity, and oxygen, so patients should preferentially be located in hospitals, although mobile critical care units are an option. Following the September 11, 2001, attacks, a mobile critical care unit was set up, but no critically ill patients were treated in this unit.[16] At this point, it is unclear how effective mobile ICUs are for treating critically ill patients following a disaster. The ED and the postanesthesia care unit are equipped to care for critically ill patients, as is the operating room (but it is likely better suited for surgical procedures). If the hospital is becoming overwhelmed, patients who are not critically ill should be moved to surge facilities, to allow for more critically ill patients to be treated in the hospital.[25] As the ED and operating room become saturated, the ICU is the next logical place for primary evaluation and resuscitation of new patients. In the Israeli experience, it has been reported that the ICU is used for the initial hospital evaluation of 11% of mass casualty victims.[46] As the ICU becomes a triage location, telemedicine consultation could improve patient triage because ICU physicians and nurses are not as experienced with patient triage as emergency physicians, nurses, and paramedics.

Tele-ICU Monitoring

As the system becomes overburdened with critically ill patients, it becomes difficult to monitor some critically ill patients while others are requiring procedures and closer attention. Monitoring patients in the ICU becomes an incredibly burdensome task when there is an abundance of critically ill patients. Tele-ICU monitoring may provide the highest benefit of any aspect of telemedicine in the disaster setting. By leaving a patient's bedside, and having a distant care provider monitoring their physiologic signs, the treating physicians can take care of the most critically ill, while only being alerted to those patients whose status is deteriorating.

Tele-ICU monitoring in a disaster can become complex. Wireless technologies would be ideal in this setting, but transmitting multiple patients' data over large distances wirelessly with limited resources can be extremely difficult. In a completely wireless setting, sensor nodes could be placed on the patients to monitor physiologic parameters, which can include telemetry, oxygen saturation, and temperature. Some patients may require more monitoring than others and some forms of monitoring may be less useful in others, so using the fewest number of sensor nodes possible decreases the risk of interference. Some environments may be wet, hot, or cold, so the sensor nodes need to be made of resilient materials. These wireless sensor nodes can then be connected to a personal control unit, which is a portable electronic device with built-in Bluetooth, Wi-Fi, mobile, and/or satellite technology to transmit data over larger distances to remote stations to collect and store data. Smartphones may be the ideal personal control unit, especially if they are equipped with satellite technology to transmit data to remote personal computers. Once the data are transmitted to a remote station, which is typically a medical center, they can then be monitored from this location or transmitted using the Internet or other more standard modes of telecommunication to a remote telemedicine provider for monitoring.[2]

Disaster Emergency Logistic Telemedicine Advanced Satellites System

The Disaster Emergency Logistic Telemedicine Advanced Satellites System (DELTASS) project was funded by the European Space Agency to create an organized telemedicine system to respond to a disaster. It provides one example of telemedicine's role in response to different phases of disaster medicine. After a disaster, a country or organization decides to provide support and deploys a mobile team, which includes search and rescue teams with portable telephones, first aid medical teams with portable telemedicine workstations, and ambulance services also with portable telemedicine workstations. These mobile teams are tracked by global positioning system satellites, and they can communicate and transmit data back to a permanent center via satellite. The permanent center is typically located outside the disaster zone in the country providing support, allowing for a quicker response because a medical field hospital within the disaster zone takes time to organize. The permanent center can also communicate with one or more reference hospitals, which are located nearby but outside the disaster area. Because the reference hospital and permanent center are located outside the disaster area, they are able to communicate by land-based telecommunications systems. Once the medical field hospital is established, communication with the reference hospital is established through VSAT satellites, which can then transfer all the information regarding the mobile teams to the reference hospital. The medical field hospital takes over control of the mobile teams, as well as medical triage, transportation, and patient data management. The reference hospital is then available for assistance triaging, diagnosing, or providing emergent care via VSAT link, which is

Table 2
Department of homeland security national planning scenarios and the potential role of telemedicine

Scenarios	Critically Ill Patient Volume	Requirements for Critical Care	Duration of Critical Care Needs	Potential for Telemedicine
Nuclear detonation in the business district of a large city	Tens to hundreds of thousands	Blast/crush injuries, burns, bone marrow suppression, septic shock, cardiovascular collapse	Weeks to months	Risk of secondary exposure, so remote care may be necessary; radiation exposure consultation; telemedicine triage; tele-ICU monitoring
Anthrax attack during rush hour exposes 330,000 people	13,000–25,000	Pneumonia with respiratory failure, ARDS, septic shock	Days to weeks	24–96 h for relief, can provide assistance; ARDS management; tele-ICU monitoring
Pandemic influenza affecting a state with 11 million people	10,000	ARDS, pneumonia, septic shock, myocardial infarction	Weeks to months	External assistance unlikely; tele-ICU monitoring; ARDS management
Biological attack with pneumonic plague at airports, trains, stadiums	6000	Pneumonia, septic shock	Days to weeks	24–96 h for relief, can provide assistance; prevent spread to other areas from airport; infectious disease consultation; epidemiology consultation to limit spread
Chemical attack with mustard gas (blistering agent) at stadium	Hundreds to thousands	Partial thickness burns, septic shock, ARDS, upper airway obstruction, trauma secondary to trampling	Days to weeks	24–96 h for relief, can provide assistance; Burn Center consultation; bioterrorism specialist consultation

Bombing of petroleum refining plant and container ships	Hundreds	Burns, inhalation injury, blast injury, chronic respiratory exacerbations	Days to weeks	Burn Center consultation; Trauma Center consultations; tele-ICU monitoring
Chemical attack with sarin gas in several office buildings	Hundreds to thousands	Seizures, paralysis, respiratory failure, coma	Days to weeks	Telemedicine triage; bioterrorism specialist consultation
Chlorine tank explosion with chlorine gas dispersion in a large city	15,000–20,000	ARDS, pulmonary edema	Days to weeks	Tele-ICU monitoring
Earthquake magnitude 7.5 in a large city	Hundreds	Crush injuries, pulmonary contusions, renal failure	Days to weeks	Telemedicine triage; tele-ICU monitoring
Category 5 hurricane in a large city	Depends on closures of other hospitals	Trauma, sepsis, drowning, exacerbations in the chronically ill	Days	Tele-ICU monitoring, recovery
Radiologic attack: dirty bombs with cesium 137 in several major cities	Hundreds	Blast injury, radiation sickness	Days to weeks	Telemedicine triage, radiation sickness specialist consultation
Conventional explosion: truck bombs on transit system	Tens to hundreds	Head injury, blast injury, burns, multiple trauma	Days to weeks	Telemedicine triage, tele-ICU monitoring

Abbreviation: ARDS, acute respiratory distress syndrome.

Data from Jurmain JC, Blancero AJ, Geiling JA, et al. HazBot: development of a telemanipulator robot with haptics for emergency response. Am J Disaster Med 2008;3(2):87–97.

best if live video transmission is possible. Besides live teleconsultation, DELTASS also has the capability to perform live telemonitoring, telesonography, telesurgery, and interactive telemicrobiology and provide Internet access and external database consultation.[2]

Potential of Telemedicine in Treating Critically Ill Patients Following Disasters

There are many potential disaster scenarios, and the Department of Homeland Security predicted the volume of critically ill patients from multiple scenarios. These scenarios have been revised to identify potential areas for telemedicine (**Table 2**).[39]

Recovery

The subacute and chronic recovery phases following a disaster are areas in which telemedicine can be critical. Immediately after a disaster, there is often an influx of humanitarian organizations to assist in acute recovery; however, weeks to years after the disaster this support likely dwindles. As the infrastructure of the area is re-established, communicating through telemedicine becomes an easier task. The patient load also continues to be high, as critically ill patients can be stuck in health care facilities for prolonged periods, and the chronically ill lose access to their medications and medical support, leading to acute exacerbations of their disease process.[2]

The National Aeronautics and Space Administration (NASA) Spacebridge to Armenia telemedicine project exemplifies the necessity for chronic disaster recovery. As a result of the December 7, 1988, Spitak earthquake in Soviet Armenia, there were greater than 50,000 deaths and 100,000 injuries and 540,000 were left homeless.[47] Because of political issues and this being the first real telemedicine response, assistance from NASA did not begin until May 1989. Communication was possible via the spacebridge using facsimile, two-way audio, and one-way video. In total, 209 patients with complications were consulted from Armenia to the United States initially by store-and-forward telemedicine by fax of patient records followed by discussion of the cases through the spacebridge, which resulted in a change in both the diagnosis and the treatment plan 25% of the time.[42,48] There was no precedent for a telemedicine project of this magnitude at the time, and it led to an Internet-based telemedicine program, the Spacebridge-to-Russia project, which was also coordinated with NASA. Improvements in Web-based electronic medical records, teletrauma, and disaster planning were some of the successes of this system.[2]

SUMMARY

Telemedicine is a new and rapidly advancing field in health care. A large proportion of ICU care is devoted to monitoring, recognizing trends, and coordinating the care of patients with specialists, which can all be done from a remote location. Telemedicine could be used to teach less experienced surrogate providers how to care for the critically ill or as the primary method of care for the critically ill as part of a well-organized disaster plan. Although telemedicine seems to be a useful modality for the care of critically ill patients after a disaster, there is little evidence to support its widespread use. Tele-ICU is clearly a costly intervention in a disaster, and studies evaluating the cost-effectiveness and clinical benefits need to be performed if telemedicine hopes to expand its role in disaster management.

REFERENCES

1. WHO. Global Observatory for eHealth series - volume 2. WHO. Available at: http://www.who.int/goe/publications/ehealth_series_vol2/en/. Accessed May 29, 2014.

2. Latifi R, editor. Telemedicine for trauma, emergencies, and disaster management. Norwood (MA): Artech House; 2011.

3. Rosenfeld BA, Dorman T, Breslow MJ, et al. Intensive care unit telemedicine: alternate paradigm for providing continuous intensivist care. Crit Care Med 2000;28(12):3925–31.

4. Breslow MJ, Rosenfeld BA, Doerfler M, et al. Effect of a multiple-site intensive care unit telemedicine program on clinical and economic outcomes: an alternative paradigm for intensivist staffing. Crit Care Med 2004;32(1):31–8. http://dx. doi.org/10.1097/01.CCM.0000104204.61296.41.

5. Wilcox ME, Adhikari NK. The effect of telemedicine in critically ill patients: systematic review and meta-analysis. Crit Care 2012;16(4):R127. http://dx.doi.org/10. 1186/cc11429.

6. Morrison JL, Cai Q, Davis N, et al. Clinical and economic outcomes of the electronic intensive care unit: results from two community hospitals. Crit Care Med 2010;38(1):2–8. http://dx.doi.org/10.1097/CCM.0b013e3181b78fa8.

7. Nassar BS, Vaughan-Sarrazin MS, Jiang L, et al. Impact of an intensive care unit telemedicine program on patient outcomes in an integrated health care system. JAMA Intern Med 2014. http://dx.doi.org/10.1001/jamainternmed.2014.1503.

8. Reynolds HN, Sheinfeld G, Chang J, et al. The tele-intensive care unit during a disaster: seamless transition from routine operations to disaster mode. Telemed J E Health 2011;17(9):746–9. http://dx.doi.org/10.1089/tmj.2011.0046.

9. Centre for Research on the Epidemiology of Disasters. The international disaster database. Available at: www.emdat.be. Accessed October 16, 2014.

10. Guha-Sapir D. Disaster data: a balanced perspective. CRED Crunch 2010;20:1–2.

11. Bilham R. The seismic future of cities. Bull Earthquake Eng 2009;7(4):839–87. http://dx.doi.org/10.1007/s10518-009-9147-0.

12. Smith AB, Katz RW. US billion-dollar weather and climate disasters: data sources, trends, accuracy and biases. Nat Hazards 2013;67(2):387–410. http://dx.doi.org/ 10.1007/s11069-013-0566-5.

13. Department of State. The Office of Website Management, Bureau of Public Affairs. National consortium for the study of terrorism and responses to terrorism: annex of statistical information. Department of State. The Office of Website Management, Bureau of Public Affairs; 2014. Available at: http://www.state.gov/j/ct/ rls/crt/2013/224831.htm. Accessed May 24, 2014.

14. Carter S, Cox A. One 9/11 tally: $3.3 trillion. Available at: http://www.nytimes.com/ interactive/2011/09/08/us/sept-11-reckoning/cost-graphic.html?_r=0. Accessed October 16, 2014.

15. Simmons S, Alverson D, Poropatich R, et al. Applying telehealth in natural and anthropogenic disasters. Telemed J E Health 2008;14(9):968–71. http://dx.doi. org/10.1089/tmj.2008.0117.

16. Kleinpeter MA, Norman LD, Krane NK. Dialysis services in the hurricane-affected areas in 2005: lessons learned. Am J Med Sci 2006;332(5):259–63.

17. Redlener I, Reilly MJ. Lessons from Sandy — preparing health systems for future disasters. N Engl J Med 2012;367(24):2269–71. http://dx.doi.org/10.1056/ NEJMp1213486.

18. Adalja AA, Watson M, Bouri N, et al. Absorbing citywide patient surge during Hurricane Sandy: a case study in accommodating multiple hospital evacuations. Ann Emerg Med 2014. http://dx.doi.org/10.1016/j.annemergmed.2013.12.010.

19. Cushman JG, Pachter HL, Beaton HL. Two New York City hospitals' surgical response to the September 11, 2001, terrorist attack in New York City. J Trauma 2003;54(1):147–55.

20. De Ceballos JP, Turégano-Fuentes F, Perez-Diaz D, et al. 11 March 2004: the terrorist bomb explosions in Madrid, Spain–an analysis of the logistics, injuries sustained and clinical management of casualties treated at the closest hospital. Crit Care 2005;9(1):104–11. http://dx.doi.org/10.1186/cc2995.

21. Aylwin CJ, König TC, Brennan NW, et al. Reduction in critical mortality in urban mass casualty incidents: analysis of triage, surge, and resource use after the London bombings on July 7, 2005. Lancet 2006;368(9554):2219–25. http://dx.doi.org/10.1016/S0140-6736(06)69896-6.

22. Balch D. Developing a national inventory of telehealth resources for rapid and effective emergency medical care: a white paper developed by the American telemedicine association emergency preparedness and response special interest group. Telemed J E Health 2008;14(6):606–10. http://dx.doi.org/10.1089/tmj.2007.0127.

23. Yu JN, Brock TK, Mecozzi DM, et al. Future connectivity for disaster and emergency point of care. Point Care 2010;9(4):185–92. http://dx.doi.org/10.1097/POC.0b013e3181fc95ee.

24. Rashvand HF, Traver Salcedo V, Monton Sanchez E, et al. Ubiquitous wireless telemedicine. IET Commun 2008;2(2):237–54.

25. Kudo D, Furukawa H, Nakagawa A, et al. Reliability of telecommunications systems following a major disaster: survey of secondary and tertiary emergency institutions in Miyagi prefecture during the acute phase of the 2011 Great East Japan earthquake. Prehosp Disaster Med 2014;29(02):204–8. http://dx.doi.org/10.1017/S1049023X14000119.

26. Bostick NA, Subbarao I, Burkle FM, et al. Disaster triage systems for large-scale catastrophic events. Disaster Med Public Health Prep 2008;2(Suppl S1):S35–9. http://dx.doi.org/10.1097/DMP.0b013e3181825a2b.

27. Available at: http://www.un-spider.org/knowledge-base/health-support-guides/pre-hospital-application-telemedicine-acute-onset-disaster-situations-matthew. Accessed February 3, 2015.

28. Jenkins JL, McCarthy ML, Sauer LM, et al. Mass-casualty triage: time for an evidence-based approach. Prehosp Disaster Med 2008;23(1):3–8.

29. Garner A, Lee A, Harrison K, et al. Comparative analysis of multiple-casualty incident triage algorithms. Ann Emerg Med 2001;38(5):541–8. http://dx.doi.org/10.1067/mem.2001.119053.

30. Wallis LA, Carley S. Comparison of paediatric major incident primary triage tools. Emerg Med J 2006;23(6):475–8. http://dx.doi.org/10.1136/emj.2005.032672.

31. Haskins PA, Ellis DG, Mayrose J. Predicted utilization of emergency medical services telemedicine in decreasing ambulance transports. Prehosp Emerg Care 2002;6(4):445–8.

32. Mathews KA, Elcock MS, Furyk JS. The use of telemedicine to aid in assessing patients prior to aeromedical retrieval to a tertiary referral centre. J Telemed Telecare 2008;14(6):309–14. http://dx.doi.org/10.1258/jtt.2008.080417.

33. Tsai SH, Kraus J, Wu HR, et al. The effectiveness of video-telemedicine for screening of patients requesting emergency air medical transport (EAMT). J Trauma 2007;62(2):504–11. http://dx.doi.org/10.1097/01.ta.0000219285.08974.45.

34. Sejersten M, Sillesen M, Hansen PR, et al. Effect on treatment delay of prehospital teletransmission of 12-lead electrocardiogram to a cardiologist for immediate triage and direct referral of patients with ST-segment elevation acute myocardial infarction to primary percutaneous coronary intervention. Am J Cardiol 2008;101(7):941–6. http://dx.doi.org/10.1016/j.amjcard.2007.11.038.

35. Kyle E, Aitken P, Elcock M, et al. Use of telehealth for patients referred to a retrieval service: timing, destination, mode of transport, escort level and patient care. J Telemed Telecare 2012;18(3):147–50. http://dx.doi.org/10.1258/jtt.2012. SFT106.
36. Meade B, Barnett P. Emergency care in a remote area using interactive video technology: a study in prehospital telemedicine. J Telemed Telecare 2002;8(2): 115–7.
37. Okumura T, Suzuki K, Fukuda A, et al. The Tokyo subway sarin attack: disaster management, Part 1: community emergency response. Acad Emerg Med 1998;5(6):613–7. http://dx.doi.org/10.1111/j.1553-2712.1998.tb02470.x.
38. Burke RV, Berg BM, Vee P, et al. Using robotic telecommunications to triage pediatric disaster victims. J Pediatr Surg 2012;47(1):221–4. http://dx.doi.org/10. 1016/j.jpedsurg.2011.10.046.
39. Jurmain JC, Blancero AJ, Geiling JA, et al. HazBot: development of a telemanipulator robot with haptics for emergency response. Am J Disaster Med 2008; 3(2):87–97.
40. Ferreira FL, Bota DP, Bross A, et al. Serial evaluation of the SOFA score to predict outcome in critically ill patients. JAMA 2001;286(14):1754–8.
41. Devereaux AV, Dichter JR, Christian MD, et al. Definitive care for the critically ill during a disaster: a framework for allocation of scarce resources in mass critical care: from a Task Force For Mass Critical Care summit meeting, January 26–27, 2007, Chicago, IL. Chest 2008;133(5 Suppl):51S–66S. http://dx.doi.org/10.1378/ chest.07-2693.
42. White DB, Katz MH, Luce JM, et al. Who should receive life support during a public health emergency? Using ethical principles to improve allocation decisions. Ann Intern Med 2009;150(2):132–8.
43. Corcoran SP, Niven AS, Reese JM. Critical care management of major disasters: a practical guide to disaster preparation in the intensive care unit. J Intensive Care Med 2012;27(1):3–10. http://dx.doi.org/10.1177/0885066610393639.
44. Christian MD, Devereaux AV, Dichter JR, et al. Definitive care for the critically ill during a disaster: current capabilities and limitations: from a Task Force For Mass Critical Care summit meeting, January 26–27, 2007, Chicago, IL. Chest 2008;133(5 Suppl):8S–17S. http://dx.doi.org/10.1378/chest.07-2707.
45. Devereaux A, Christian MD, Dichter JR, et al. Summary of suggestions from the Task Force For Mass Critical Care summit, January 26–27, 2007. Chest 2008; 133(5 Suppl):1S–7S. http://dx.doi.org/10.1378/chest.08-0649.
46. Avidan V, Hersch M, Spira RM, et al. Civilian hospital response to a mass casualty event: the role of the intensive care unit. J Trauma 2007;62(5):1234–9. http://dx. doi.org/10.1097/01.ta.0000210483.04535.e0.
47. Doarn CR, Merrell RC. Spacebridge to armenia: a look back at its impact on telemedicine in disaster response. Telemed J E Health 2011;17(7):546–52. http://dx. doi.org/10.1089/tmj.2010.0212.
48. Houtchens BA, Clemmer TP, Holloway HC, et al. Telemedicine and international disaster response: medical consultation to Armenia and Russia via a Telemedicine Spacebridge. Prehosp Disaster Med 1993;8(1):57–66.

Increasing Quality Through Telemedicine in the Intensive Care Unit

Thomas H. Kalb, MD[a,b],*

KEYWORDS

- Performance improvement • Process indicator • Outcome indicator
- Culture of safety • Team building • TeleICU data management
- Cross-sectional analysis • Longitudinal analysis

KEY POINTS

- Quality Process Improvement in the ICU requires a system for data collection and analysis, dedicated resources, and a culture of safety that drives the process.
- The TeleICU platform is well equipped to provide all of the elements of successful Quality Process Improvement.
- Hurdles to the successful implementation of a TeleICU directed Quality Process Improvement include loss of data fidelity, strains on resources, and barriers across the TeleICU environment that hinder the development of a culture of safety.
- A completed Quality Process Improvement initiative to direct ventilator rounds across a TeleICU platform is described in some detail so as to point out features that lead to success and possible strategies to overcome the hurdles.

INTRODUCTION

This article explores the hypothesis that a telemedicine intensive care unit (TeleICU) platform is uniquely suited to facilitate quality performance improvement (PI). At the same time, this article also addresses some of the substantial hurdles to overcome that may limit the effectiveness of a TeleICU platform to achieve PI objectives. Lastly, this article describes in some detail the author's experience with an ongoing PI project to improve ventilator management conducted via a TeleICU hub interacting with 11 geographically dispersed ICUs. Using this example to illustrate the concepts, the author hopes to shed some realistic light on the successes and lessons learned so as to generate best-practice guidelines for TeleICU-directed PI initiatives.

Disclosure: No extramural support.
[a] Advance ICUcare Medical Group, 747 Third Avenue, 28th Floor, New York, NY 10017, USA;
[b] Department of Medicine, North Shore/LIJ Hofstra School of Medicine, Manhassat, NY, USA
* Advance ICUcare Medical Group, 747 Third Avenue, 28th Floor, New York, NY 10017.
E-mail address: tkalb@icumedicine.com

Crit Care Clin 31 (2015) 257–273
http://dx.doi.org/10.1016/j.ccc.2014.12.005
0749-0704/15/$ – see front matter © 2015 Elsevier Inc. All rights reserved.

How Is a Telemedicine Intensive Care Unit Platform Aligned with a Quality Performance Improvement Mission?

PI activities can be defined as any systematic, data-driven, clinically focused program that is intended to improve a defined set of processes or outcomes on a defined cohort of patients, often focused on a particular disease or illness.[1] For example, in the case of ventilator-associated pneumonia, a *process indicator* might measure the timeliness, accuracy, or incidence of a targeted activity, such as the implementation of appropriate antibiotics, whereas *outcome indicators* measure clinical events, such as the incidence of worsening lung injury scores in patients requiring more than 48 hours of mechanical ventilation.

In general, quality PI activities are conducted daily, folded into clinical activities, often with dedicated stakeholders but almost always with participation of the clinical team. In the ICU setting, PI programs have taken many guises and have focused on a diverse array of clinical activities. Often, ICU PI initiatives stem from an effort to bolster adherence to best-practice guidelines that have been vetted and endorsed by expert panels, such as the Surviving Sepsis guidelines promoted by the Society of Critical Care Medicine (SCCM) or the standards for deep vein thrombosis (DVT) prophylaxis as published periodically by the American College of Chest Physicians. In other instances, successful PI initiatives are driven by more local issues, such as tackling throughput bottlenecks, to identify and overcome local dynamics that limit efficiency and successful patient triage.[2]

TeleICU is conducive to quality PI by virtue of the natural alignment of the TeleICU basic tool kit with the required PI implementation package. In all successful PI initiatives, irrespective of the particular focus, 3 domains have been cited as being critical; these same domains are also integral components of most TeleICU systems.[3] These characteristic components can be summarized under the headings of *Good data, Dedicated resources*, and *Team building for a culture of safety*.

Good data

The aphorism *you can't improve what you can't measure* is so often cited in quality PI circles as to be a widely accepted maxim. Having said that, there is no greater challenge in the critical care arena than to capture meaningful data that can be brought to bear on PI objectives. The challenges are daunting, not the least of which stems from the complex physiology of critically ill patients and the heterogeneous mix of disease states that come under the critical care umbrella. With so much going on, so much being measured, and at so rapid a pace, with so few resources available to dedicate to collecting data, information overload and lapses are a given. Simply stated, TeleICU offers a unique solution to provide a comprehensive, prospective, real-time accruing database.

Of the products available to provide TeleICU monitoring services, the proprietary software package by Philips VISICU presently enjoys market dominance and serves as the model to illustrate PI alignment in this article.

The data management software package eCareManager (Philips VISICU, Baltimore, MD) that is the center post of the Philips VISICU platform provides the TeleICU clinician with a uniform display of clinical information by culling multiple sources of electronic medical record (EMR) stream into an organized critical care flow sheet for each patient. This organization is critical to the day-to-day management of large volumes of patients from diverse settings by providing a uniform and concise clinical summary. At the same time, this same information that streams into the TeleICU center for clinical use is also downloaded into a reducible and mineable database that is collected by the software proprietor and used to prepare quarterly performance reports.

Several features of this database make it particularly suitable to PI application. Firstly, the database is anonymized in that all information leaving the clinical realm is stripped of Protected Health Information [PHI] identifiers and is secured behind HIPAA (Health Insurance Portability and Accountability Act) protected firewalls. This feature can help to overcome Institutional Review Board requirements and permit unfettered PI activities and of course to protect patients' rights and privacy.

Secondly, the process is predominantly automatic; most of the information is obtained by direct interface with electronic systems. Yet certain qualitative clinical information may not be available by electronic means. The eCareManager system has addressed this with the opportunity for manual or assisted (drop-down menu) entry to supplement the automated data accrual. For example, TeleICU personnel may generate a list of admitting diagnoses based on clinical criteria, for example, to identifying acute respiratory distress syndrome (ARDS) as a cause of acute respiratory failure.

No additional personnel are required to transfer information from the clinical site to the database because the single-use pathway serves both clinical and data accrual purposes. There are also no data omissions or time lapses because of availability of this service on weekends or nighttime. Thus, incumbent on the routine clinical operations of the TeleICU monitoring system, the PI team is afforded with a trove of data without additional efforts or resource.

Thirdly, specific rule sets and censoring filters limit spurious outliers/electronic errors that provide a layer of confidence in the measured values. Error analysis is codified in a user's handbook created by the proprietary-based management team, where terms are defined, and the analytical method transparently described.

Fourthly, the number of data points can be quite large, depending on the number of centers that are engaged in the PI activity. With multiple ICUs tied to one TeleICU center, large numbers of patients and countable events can be incorporated into the project, allowing for a foreshortened timeline to tests of significance and power analyses that realistically predict large sample numbers. Moreover, the entire proprietary database is large—massive really—as a result of the Phillips system's dominance in market share for TeleICU application, so that platform-wide comparative analysis is shared with all TeleICU providers and predictive scoring tools have a very robust denominator.

This sizable cohort of the entire eICU database has generated its own predictive model for acuity and prediction scoring for readmission that has been tested and validated on million-plus robust cohorts.

However, just having a big database may not be adequate to cull information that permits process improvement endeavors. It is one thing to obtain a data point (eg, ventilator duration), but without a benchmark by which to make comparison this single piece of information may lack the dimension required for performance analysis and improvement that is matched to a standard. In other words, in order to best assess any process or outcome, it is essential to have a starting point and a measured end point; but it can be most informative to compare these points with a validated and external benchmark.

The TeleICU proprietary service reports benchmarked data on a variety of process and outcome indicators. A quarterly report is generated for each participating ICU, and comparative analysis is prepared for each center that shows performance characteristics relative to all other participating centers. Included in the quarterly benchmark reports are adherence to DVT prophylaxis, stress ulcer prophylaxis, glycemic control parameters, and low tidal volume protective lung ventilation.

For certain outcomes, the Acute Physiology and Chronic Health Evaluation (APACHE) IV regression equations are used to analyze data residing in the eCareManager database. These APACHE IV scores are used to generate individual patient outcome predictions for days of mechanical ventilation, ICU mortality, and length of stay (LOS). The actual outcomes are compared with predicted outcomes as mortality, LOS, and ventilator day ratios for each ICU. Then individual outcome ratios are combined to generate the mean outcome ratios. Philips VISICU provides a Benchmark Report User's Guide to the TeleICU center that provides an overview, definitions, and details of the preparation methods of the data.

In sum, TeleICU provides a rich database source that is large, robust, automated, benchmarked, and focused on important processes and outcomes. In many ways, the greatest hurdle in process improvement efforts to create a data management infrastructure is done for you and folded into the working apparatus of the TeleICU service.

Dedicated resources

Even with the tantalizing potential of big data offered by TeleICU, valuable information may just sit there unless resources are dedicated to their creative and focused utilization. Dedicating time, attention, personnel, and dollars in a sustained manner is a great existential challenge in the PI world, because all agree that the primary task of all ICUs is to serve the clinical needs of critically ill patients. What this also means is that all other tasks, including PI initiatives, must necessarily take a subsidiary role, particularly in the world of limited resources that is the reality of health care delivery.

The challenge of doing more with less, of allocating scarce resources to PI, requires new solutions; TeleICU resource utilization may be part of those solutions. The additional TeleICU clinical staff and support personnel can be a powerful resource to reinforce bedside team efforts to plan, actuate, sustain, and analyzing process improvement initiatives.

The TeleICU team structure varies in composition and job description, though in general, all systems have adopted a pyramidal hierarchy so that for each intensivist physician, there may be several advanced practice providers, critical care registered nurse (CCRN), and data specialists that perform separate tasks. Combining with the bedside services, this additional manpower may provide the breathing room necessary to free up resources to conduct the planning, executing, and analysis of PI initiatives.

Combining manpower resources with 24-hour monitoring may permit for dedicated time and personnel who concentrate on PI activities. One example in the author's particular TeleICU service is a targeted program that directs protocol and resources to monitor and manage glycemic control.

Team building for a culture of safety

TeleICU practice implementation may enhance the development of a culture of safety and must incorporate team building with bedside services in order for successful performance. Models of TeleICU vary by environment, structure, and protocol, with reported outcome measures that differ. However, with regard to those manifestations of culture that drive PI, almost all TeleICU endeavors share a common focus, enhanced by automated TeleICU systems, to monitor and enhance best-practice adherence.[4–6]

Cultural awareness of safety and a team-building ethos is critical to successful PI initiatives in the ICU. For any project to be sustained, stakeholders must convey to the entire health care team in the ICU a culture of safety, inclusion, and empowerment, wherein each individual buys into the concept of the shared responsibility for patient care delivery and PI.

Although widely touted that team building is crucial, it is equally acknowledged to be a great challenge to ingenuity and resources to capture the spirit and sustain the attention of busy caregivers and even more so to nurture and sustain the qualities of team effort that are often resisted or dissipate with time.

Models of team building in ICU settings emphasize the need to put systems in place that focus on commitment to multidisciplinary participation, respecting and acknowledging the contributions of various members of the clinical team. The need for vigilance and daily practice patterns that put principle into practice are equally emphasized, in that reiteration and reward in the form of periodic sharing of data with all team members helps to demonstrate payoff to all participants.

What Are the Major Hurdles to Overcome in Telemedicine Intensive Care Unit–Leveraged Performance Improvement Activities?

Not-so-good data

The automated database requires attention and support to provide reliable data. Processes that are not captured or outcomes that are incompletely or inaccurately entered into the database will deteriorate data fidelity. There are several ways in which the electronic automated downloading of data can be confounded. For example, some components of EMR may be entered manually. One example might be ventilator settings coupled to an arterial blood gas (ABG) measurement; thus, the reliability of values derived from such entries may be susceptible to mistakes and omissions.

Secondly, data that originate from more than one ICU often demonstrate wide practice variation. Therefore, combining data from multiple centers may generate mean baseline data with a large standard deviation. When each ICU has its own starting point, then this can contribute to broad error estimates that dilute the ability to detect relevant change. Therefore, tests of significance may be frustratingly difficult to achieve given the large error inherent in such calculations.

Thirdly, many of the outcome elements that are provided by the proprietary database are reported as ratios linked to the APACHE IV score. Thus, the accuracy of APACHE IV scoring is a critical feature that requires attention in any PI endeavor that uses these measures. Uniformity among scoring depends not only on automated access to laboratory data but also to vital sign record and qualitative assessment profile, such as listing chronic comorbidities and accurate description of admitting diagnoses. In order to work toward uniformity, consistency, and validity in data entry that requires clinical personnel, orientation to details of APACHE IV scoring methods and maintenance of training is required.

Fourthly, disparate centers with a different patient mix, distinct service providers and personnel, and clinical frameworks that vary provide a unique challenge to avoiding bias and random drift. With so many variables at play, it can be a daunting task to assign causation to any outcome and to assign meaning or design to any process improvement. The classic clinical research model of well-matched cohorts with single exposures and unambiguous quantitative end points is essentially unheard of in the TeleICU environment.

At a minimum, it is prudent to avoid falling into an unwarranted assumption of causation with any observed difference. In essence, the concern with TeleICU data sets that accrue multicenter data from uncontrolled multiparameter-based observations is that TeleICU data sets are attempting to compare proverbial apples with oranges.

If greater rigor is desired or if PI efforts are coupled with planned submission for publication, then innovative statistical solutions may need to be brought to bear on the database analysis.

To better control for such dynamic changes and to better capture the effect of the process improvement intervention, it may be necessary to overlay process control analysis using control charts specially designed to capture the essence of PI-derived changes over time.[7] The principal advantage of using control chart methodology is to distinguish between so-called common cause variation (chance) and special cause variation (assignable). Methodology applied to process control helps to account for variation, such as case mix and other population changes that may vary between data collection intervals and introduce bias in the observations.

By adopting process control analysis, the author hopes to better clarify that the changes detected were indeed durable and dependent on process improvement initiatives using a TeleICU platform rather than a general shift in patient population or practice pattern over time.

Strains on resources
Despite the importance of a PI mission, all clinical personnel on both sides of this equation are being asked to do more with less. The extra resources added through TeleICU services have a primary monitoring and intervention role that is a priority. Therefore, the ability to accomplish PI tasks in a continuous and meaningful way is always in tension with the provision of primary care responsibilities. The ambitions and goals put forth by stakeholders must take this limitation most seriously when designing process improvement initiatives. The most important way to manage resources is to combine processes that contribute to both process improvement while at the same time provide for clinical care.

Not surprisingly, variations in TeleICU resource utilization have resulted in a broad range of putative impacts, with claims of substantial as well as no measurable impact on ICU outcomes. For example, in a care model format of low resource utilization, whereby a large fraction of bedside physicians chose to contract only for limited Tele-ICU engagement (ie, only to intercede in cardiopulmonary arrest or ongoing emergency), the impact of TeleICU services on important outcome measures, such as mortality and LOS, were not detected.[8–10] Conversely, it has been speculated that in settings where high-intensity 24-7 intensivist services are already in place, the additive effect of TeleICU services would be substantially muted. In essence, the technological platform afforded by TeleICU, like any new technology, has variable applications and impact that seems quite sensitive to process and environment.[10]

Bridging culture: home team versus visitors
Because TeleICU services are offsite, not physically present in the ICU, and are manned by personnel with loose affiliation, there are often substantial issues of trust and cooperation that must be overcome in a programmatic manner to lead to an effective combined-forces effort in PI.[11] The entire TeleICU endeavor, including PI efforts, is seen through 2 distinct perspectives: the home team of each ICU and the visitor bench occupied by the TeleICU personnel. Bringing these two teams into a cooperative posture always requires a mindful and empathetic approach to overcome differences to the mutual benefit to patients and caregivers.

However, because disparate programs may be tethered together through a central TeleICU hub, along with the functional alignment with process improvement intrinsic to the platform, success depends on overcoming disparity, differences, and local factors among ICU environments. These intrinsic differences compete with attempts to unify practice patterns, because TeleICU linked programs may manifest vastly different baseline characteristics, and local factors such as manpower, patient mix and other pressures may impose distinct barriers to faithful implementation of centralized initiatives. The urgent day to day critical care needs can submerge even the best of intentions for process improvement into a competitive struggle for access to data, resources and the cultural imperatives necessary for successful initiatives.

Putting It All Together: the Author's Experience with a Quality Performance Improvement Initiative Conducted via Telemedicine Intensive Care Unit Platform

The author conducted a retrospective, population-based, cross-sectional, and longitudinal analysis before and after implementation of a quality PI project to improve the process and outcomes via TeleICU-directed daily bedside ventilator rounds.[12] This PI project was coupled with a retrospective analysis to examine the effect of exposure to TeleICU-directed ventilator rounds on one process and 2 outcome indicators. The process examined was adherence to a low tidal volume benchmark, and the outcome measures were ventilator duration ratio (VDR) and ICU mortality ratio.[13]

Despite the basic knowledge that low tidal volumes improve outcomes, many other limitations to adherence have been cited. Prominently cited limitations are diagnostic uncertainty for acute lung injury (ALI)/ARDS, a poor estimate or calculation of the Pao_2/fraction of inspired oxygen (Fio_2) (P/F) ratio, and predicted body weight (PBW)–based tidal volume. In addition, there seem to be organizational and management challenges to its implementation, including the absence of an effective protocol to target and monitor adherence and a lack of time or structure to bring together dedicated staff. Finally there is practitioner bias that excludes eligible patients borne out of a perception of physiologic worsening, symptom burden, and increased sedative need associated with lung-protective ventilation (LPV) settings despite evidence to the contrary.[14–16]

In this regard, TeleICU platforms may augment bedside adherence to ventilator benchmarks through automated calculation and display of P/F ratios, PBW-based tidal volumes, as well as by virtue of additional monitoring staff with a process improvement focus.

There were 3 phases of this process improvement project. Firstly, the data, resources, and team-building components were put in place. The PI team added data collection elements that overlay on the basic software package; resources were garnered; and training, orientation, and team-building activities reached across from the TeleICU center to the bedside partners. Secondly, the actual ventilator round activities were phased in over 2 years in 11 different ICU centers. Thirdly, the data were analyzed to assess the process and outcome indicators, which were brought back to the bedside team for reiterative process improvement reinforcement.

How Was the Telemedicine Intensive Care Unit Center Environment Organized to Conduct Process Improvement?

As described earlier, this study was conducted by an independent TeleICU practice using Philips VISICU-licensed eCareManager platform. The author's practice provides continuous patient surveillance, with all patients evaluated on admission by board-certified intensivists and followed daily by TeleICU CCRNs with intensivist involvement for clinical matters of importance. Activities include acute management as well as structured process and workflow to ensure best-practice compliance, with particular emphasis on DVT prophylaxis, glycemic control, stress ulcer prophylaxis, and low tidal volume ventilation.

The TeleICU practitioners worked in a team assigned to a cluster of hospitals, with each practitioner stationed at a multiscreen monitor array. Clinical monitoring tools that are accessible through these workstations include real-time interfaces with each hospital's information system (HIS), clinical practitioner order entry system (CPOE), radiology imaging systems, bedside monitors, as well as bedside teleconference capability.

Through eCareManager, the TeleICU practitioner can readily access individual patient data when called to intervene or conduct rounds. Imbedded capabilities include alert icons that flag all patients receiving mechanical ventilation, calculation of a P/F ratio, tidal volume in milliliter per kilogram per PBW, documentation of pulmonary mechanics, display of ventilator settings and ABG results. Orders can be entered via eCareManager, which are transmitted securely to each ICU nursing station. Alternatively, the hospital CPOE can be accessed remotely by the TeleICU intensivist in similar fashion to bedside practitioners who access CPOE and EMR through desktop stations within the ICU.

Working with Bedside Partners to Prepare the Performance Improvement Landscape

Eleven hospitals were included that subscribed to TeleICU services during both before and after ventilator rounds implementation. Participating institutions were moderate-sized community hospital ICUs from a wide geographic distribution.

Participating centers used diverse HIS/CPOE, protocols, as well as differing practice and staffing models. The ICU size ranged from 8 beds to 28 bed units. None of the centers used a fully closed-model ICU, with the most frequent model being bedside intensivist coverage limited to daytime hours and ventilator management responsibilities shared with consulting pulmonary, hospitalist services, and intensivists. Rotating family practice house staff was present in one of the ICUs.

Development of the template ventilator rounds checklist instrument and process

The established target for the clinical project was to facilitate a daily organized appraisal of proper adherence to low tidal volume ventilation in intubated patients and, when appropriate, extubation. The central organizing instrument of this process was a checklist to help ensure that TeleICU practitioners evaluated ABGs, secretions, sedation levels, PBW-based tidal volumes, and P/F ratios.

Initially these tasks and data entry were recorded on a paper checklist template. In the second year of this process, there was a transition to an electronic format for this checklist (**Fig. 1**). This electronic format was designed by TeleICU information technology personnel with automated drop-down list functionality to facilitate its completion and for the transmission of information through intranet access for all participants. This format also allowed for automated database entry and retrieval.

Building the Team: Establishing a Shared Vision for a Culture of Safety

Ventilator rounds were phased into practice one hospital at a time over a 2-year implementation period schematically depicted in **Fig. 2**. In preparation for implementation in each hospital, at least one meeting between TeleICU medical directors and the local physician, nursing, and respiratory therapy were devoted to ventilator rounds orientation. These meetings were held to introduce the topic of ventilator rounds and described the scope and intended purpose. These introductory meetings also provided a forum for discussion and consensus on joint goals for process improvement and familiarity and endorsement of benchmark standards as well as logistical details, such as timing of daily rounds and who would be participating. Before implementation, the TeleICU intensivist medical group was provided guidelines for conducting ventilator rounds that included the goals and agreed on benchmark guidelines for LPV and orientation to the internal checklist form.

Once initiated in a given hospital, multidisciplinary ventilator rounds occurred at set times, with daily participation of TeleICU physicians using audiovisual link and phone calls to bedside respiratory therapists and nursing personnel.

Members of the multidisciplinary team entered their observations in the ventilator rounds template. For each patient, the TeleICU nursing personnel entered the sedation level and interruption schedule. The bedside nursing personnel was contacted

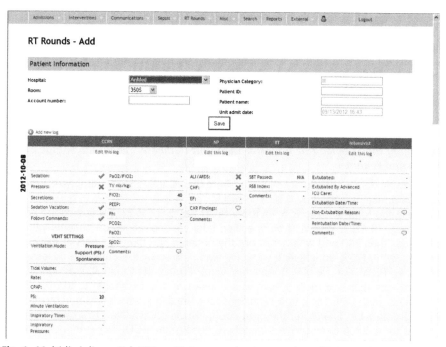

Fig. 1. Multidisciplinary TeleICU ventilator round entry template. CPAP, continuous positive airway pressure; PEEP, positive end-expiratory pressure.

by TeleICU nursing personnel to obtain information regarding secretions and airflow limitation. Midlevel personnel reviewed the vent rounds template that contains the information gathered from the electronic record, including auto-populated tidal volume per kilogram per PBW, ventilator settings, ABG, chest x-ray, and minute volume, and made an overall assessment of potential liberation readiness. When documented in the EMR, the bedside respiratory therapy notes were reviewed.

Informed by these prepopulated elements, the TeleICU intensivist then made teleconference contact with respiratory therapy and bedside nursing personnel at each intubated patient's bedside where virtual rounds were conducted. The TeleICU intensivist was free to engage the participants without script or formal talking points.

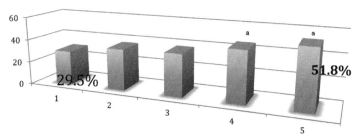

Fig. 2. Process indicator quarterly results: Improvement in adherence to low tidal volume benchmark (less than 7.5 mL/kg/PBW) for patients with ALI. This result was achieved by TeleICU-directed ventilator rounds conducted daily with 11 partner hospital ICUs. [a] $P<.001$ compared with quarter 1.

Decisions regarding liberation readiness and ventilator setting changes including tidal volume adjustments to address benchmark goals could be ordered directly by the Tel-eICU intensivist. Alternatively, based on prior agreement in some centers, the findings were treated as consultative recommendations that were then deferred to bedside practitioners for final decision making and orders. The results of ventilator rounds were accrued in the electronic record to document whether spontaneous breathing trial and tidal volume (Vt) adjustment or ventilator liberation were initiated during rounds.

Leveraging the Telemedicine Intensive Care Unit Database: Taking Advantage of the Automated Features

These study data were entirely extracted from the eCareManager database, a proprietary database managed by Philips VISICU.

Adherence to LPV is reported in the VISICU database in categories based on the percentage of ABGs drawn at prespecified tidal-volume ranges on patients with P/F ratios less than 300 and whether or not the patients had the diagnosis of ARDS. For patients with ARDS, compliance with LPV was defined by the database as less than 6.5 mL/kg/PBW. For non-ARDS patients with P/F ratios less than 300, a more liberal value of less than 7.5 mL/kg/PBW was chosen by the database as the cutoff for compliance with LPV. The cutoff definitions for compliance were stipulated by the proprietary database. Therefore, the data could not be recalculated to assign different choices for a cutoff definition that matched those of the SCCM's recent guidelines.

For example, compliance with LPV in a non-ARDS cohort was defined as

$$\text{Compliance with LPV(non ARDS)} = \frac{\# \text{ of ABG drawn with ventilator} < 7.5 \tfrac{\text{mL}}{\text{kg}} \big/ \text{PBW}}{\text{Total } \# \text{ of ABGs drawn for that hospital}} \times 100$$

The system divides the Po_2 by the Fio_2 decimal value to arrive at the oxygenation ratio and then divides the TV value in the ABG vent result by the PBW to obtain the calculated Vt, that is, Vt/PBW = calculated Vt in milliliter per kilogram per PBW. The strategy to collect TV data at the time of ABG allowed for a more accurate assessment of the adjustments that were made on individual patients, at least in part as a result of ventilator rounds interventions. Thus, an individual patient who had tidal volume adjustment could contribute data points that were initially nonadherent but were later adjusted to adherent values. Patients whose P/F ratio improved to values greater than 300 were no longer included in the analysis, though such patients might very well have continued to receive VT that were adherent to the benchmark. Data points were excluded when the height or sex was not entered, when the ABG results were incompletely entered, or when the value for TV was less than 200. The system classified patients as having ARDS when they had active diagnosis categories that included ARDS chosen by the TeleICU nurse in the admission note drop-down menu.

Ventilator duration ratio

The VDR is calculated as the number of days of mechanical ventilation per APACHE IV–predicted days of mechanical ventilation. Therefore, cohorts of patients with a VDR less than 1.0 would have been extubated before the APACHE IV prediction. Alternatively, cohorts of patients with a VDR greater than 1.0 would have done worse than expected. APACHE IV scoring is performed on the first ICU day by definition. As a result APACHE IV predicted ratios of VDR and ICU mortality ratio, all included patients required to be initiated on mechanical ventilation on APACHE IV day 1. Patients were considered ventilated by a standard routine that involved inspection of information populated within eCareManager, including the respiratory flow-sheet template, and the care plan whereby drop-down pick lists included the ventilated status. The Tele-ICU nurse entered the timing of extubation into eCareManager after corroboration of the exact time of extubation with the local bedside team. The ventilator days report that is provided by VISICU shows the number of patient stays for the quarter, then the number of stays where the patient was ventilated, total patient and ventilator days, and average and median ventilator days per patient. Units with fewer than 50 scored stays for the quarter are not included.

During the postimplementation period, a standard for defining ventilator days changed: Beginning in quarter 4 (Q4) 2011, patients with noninvasive ventilation for greater than 6 hours were added to patients counted as ventilated. Also beginning in Q4 2011, patients were considered ventilated for a day when they are ventilated for any fraction of a calendar day.

Now the Manual Labor: Taking the Proprietary Spreadsheets and Performing Cross-sectional and Longitudinal Analysis

These data from the VISICU-prepared proprietary database were then used to perform cross-sectional and longitudinal comparison of end points. As depicted in **Fig. 2**, the preimplementation quarter data from Q4 2009 were compared with the postimplementation quarter (Q3 2011) that occurred after all centers had participated in at least 3 quarters of ventilator rounds, and a follow-up cross-sectional analysis was calculated for the most recent quarter for which data were available for analysis (Q1 2012).

Because such before-and-after cross-sectional analysis may be hampered by unmeasured changes in practice across the broad implementation interval, the author next performed longitudinal analysis whereby he examined the individual hospital results shown here before and for the subsequent 3 quarters after the implementation for that individual hospital. Then mean data for each quarter were combined for all centers, treating the mean percentage of adherence as a continuous variable for statistical analysis.

Ventilator duration ratio and intensive care unit mortality

VDR and ICU mortality were reported as population means. Tests of significance to compare preimplementation and postimplementation mean values and longitudinal quarterly differences were performed by the 2-tailed student's T test.

Low tidal volume adherence

The determination of height, sex, tidal volume, and calculated tidal volume in units of milliliter per kilogram per PBW was recorded automatically at the time of each blood gas analysis within eCareManager. The database reports adherence to the low tidal volume benchmark as a binary standard, reporting percent adherence based on a VISICU-defined benchmark of less than 7.5 mL/kg/PBW for a P/F ratio less than 300 and less than 6.5 mL/kg/PBW for those patients in whom the diagnostic code for ARDS was entered into eCareManager within the first 24 hours of ICU admission. These individual determinations at each blood gas determination were then aggregated for each ICU and reported as adherent percentage of the entire ABG sample for the ICU population.

Cross-sectional analysis combined weighted means of the entire 11 hospital adherence data to perform test of significant difference by 2 × 2 table analysis using the Fisher exact test. Tests of significance for longitudinal analysis comparing quarterly mean adherence fraction were performed by 2-tailed student's T test.

What Was the Measured Impact of the Performance Improvement Project on Process and Outcome?

Low tidal volume adherence

In patients with a P/F ratio less than 300, the percentage adherent to Vt less than 7.5 mL/kg/ PBW improved from 34.0% to 47.5% (P<.001; n = 3813) in cross-sectional analysis after implementation of TeleICU ventilator rounds, and this was sustained into the most recent quarter (52.0% [P<.001; Q1/2012; n = 3272]) (see **Fig. 2**).

Percent adherence improved in 10 out of the 11 participating hospitals. The author noted that the one center without improvement suspended ventilator rounds soon after implementation, though this center continued to receive quarterly benchmark reports on these measures.

By longitudinal analysis, the author observed an incremental and significant improvement by the third quarter after implementation overall from 29.5% preimplementation to 44.9% adherence by the end of a year of ventilator rounds, and this was sustained over the most recent quarter (51.8%, P<.003). Also, the author observed no difference between centers that started ventilator rounds in an early versus late implementation period.

In the subset of patients with documented ARDS/ALI on admission, Vt less than 6.5 mL/kg/PBW improved from 23.3% to 37.0% (P<.005). However, ARDS/ALI as an admitting diagnosis was incompletely and inconsistently applied without a validated instrument. This situation was likely a result of the requirement for the TeleICU admitting nurse to enter the diagnosis by drop-down menu entry to capture this clinical entity. Additionally ARDS developing after the 24 hours is not captured by this assessment by APACHE-stipulated data entry interval limited to first APACHE IV day. ARDS diagnosis was more commonly applied in the post-implementation cross-sectional data collection interval. This increase seems to result from retraining and orientation of nursing staff to consensus definition and to the proper use of a scroll-down diagnostic menu to designate ARDS as a diagnostic category rather than changing prevalence of ARDS during this interval.

Ventilator duration ratio

The mean VDR changed from 1.08 to 0.92, and this represented a significant mean −15.8% decrease after vent rounds implementation (P<.04) (**Fig. 3**). However, the baseline VDR range of 0.66 to 1.90 reflected wide practice variation and led to a sizable standard error and nonsignificant change in absolute VDR. There were no significant differences between APACHE IV scores among participating centers (mean preimplementation quarter APACHE range 47.0–53.3; P = not significant [NS]) and no longitudinal change in mean APACHE IV scores across all centers over the sampled cross-sectional intervals (mean quarterly APACHE IV score across all centers 51.1, 51.3, and 51.0 for preimplementation, Q3/2011, and Q1/2012, respectively, P = NS).

Intensive care unit mortality

The ICU mortality ratio demonstrated longitudinal improvement that reached significance after the second quarter postimplementation (0.94 vs 0.8, 0.73, and 0.67 postimplementation) (**Fig. 4**). Because these ratios are performed using APACHE IV predictions, the mortality ratio consistently reflects the severity of illness and comorbidity characteristics of patients across the longitudinal comparison time points.

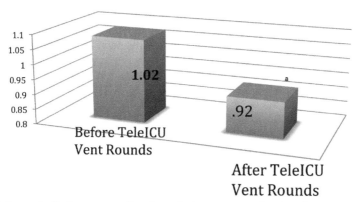

Fig. 3. Outcome indicator cross-sectional results: Improvement in VDR after implementation of TeleICU-directed ventilator rounds conducted daily with 11 partner hospital ICUs. Expressed as a ratio of ventilator days/APACHE IV predicted ventilator days. [a] Represents 15.8% reduction $P<.05$.

What Were the Effective Components of Telemedicine Intensive Care Unit Systems That Enhanced This Performance Improvement Project

The unique feature of this process was the virtual forum designed by the TeleICU service to supplement the bedside process improvement activities. This forum served as a semiautomated shared data-entry portal that was a resource for a multidisciplinary team that consisted of the TeleICU clinical team and bedside personnel. Coupled with specific workflow dedicated to ventilator management, these TeleICU ventilator rounds were brought to bear on joint decision making even when all stakeholders could not regularly meet together at every bedside for this purpose.

In contradistinction to other studies of TeleICU impact, this study was not a before-and-after comparison of the overall effect of TeleICU implementation, but rather was conducted well after the initiation of TeleICU services. By introducing ventilator rounds in the framework of an established TeleICU service relationship, the effect of this focused process improvement initiative could be detected above and beyond that of the multiple and complex dynamic changes that accompany TeleICU service initiation.

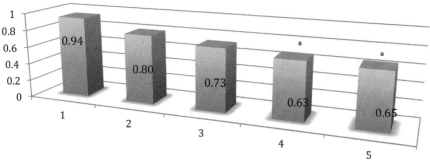

Fig. 4. Outcome indicator (quarterly results): Improvement in ICU mortality ratio (ICU mortality/APACHE IV-predicted mortality) after implementation of TeleICU-directed ventilator rounds conducted daily with 11 partner hospital ICUs. [a] $P<.04$ compared with Q1.

Although it has been reported that patients with ALI cared for in closed-model ICUs are more likely to receive lower Vt and less likely to receive high Vt, in this study, the observed improvement in process and outcome was seen across ICU settings using diverse management structures.[17] The impact was similar in ICUs managed in semi-closed models with dedicated intensivist coverage as well as in ICUs using low-intensity models wherein individual practitioners did not engage in daily multidisciplinary rounds. Thus, the observed benefit of this process was not limited to those sites with a receptive team in place and the benefits were not relegated to those sites that had no preexisting bedside counterpart.

The incremental improvement in LPV adherence over time was shown to be durable. This durability may suggest that, by the daily reiteration of this process, a modulation of potentially ingrained patterns of behavior and culture was one possible benefit of TeleICU rounds. That improved adherence to benchmarks was possible across the range of low and high preperformers suggests that opportunities for successful PI was available to a wide range of preexisting conditions. Additionally, the incremental improvement suggests that the observed change was not the result of preimplementation meetings alone, where best-practice goals were discussed and targets agreed on, because the impact of such single reinforcement meetings would be expected to dissipate with time, not to accrue benefit over the ensuing year.

The magnitude of improvement seen in this novel virtual process is consistent with previously reported bedside process improvement initiatives that dedicate additional manpower and process to efforts to improve ventilator bundle adherence. A common theme in both virtual and bedside PI efforts is that daily reinforcement, method consistency, and periodic educational initiatives to reinforce principles and provide feedback to bedside providers are key components that bring successful and durable improvement in LPV and ventilator bundle adherence.[18,19] One advantage of TeleICU-directed ventilator rounds in this study is the enhanced capacity to leverage scarce manpower and provide dedicated and consistent resource allocation that may not be available in all centers. TeleICU database results were shared with each center on a quarterly basis, providing the bedside practitioners with their individual center performance, and this helped reinforce team building and contributed to improved performance.

What Were the Biggest Limitations of Reaching Across the Telemedicine Intensive Care Unit Divide to Affect Change at the Bedside?

There are several limitation of the data obtained from this project. The retrospective-observational nature of the data analysis does not permit direct causal association of any of the observations, but rather may help to support the generation of hypothesis-testing studies in the future to examine which elements of the initiative, if any, could be responsible for the observed improvement in performance and outcome.

Indeed, the exposure to daily ventilator rounds may have impacted on process and outcome measures by an aggregate effect of multiple components. As an exposure, ventilator rounds were directed toward best practices including but not limited to low tidal volume adherence. The scope of ventilator rounds included the process of judging liberation readiness, sedation adjustments, initiation of spontaneous breathing trials and ventilator mode, and setting adjustments. Given these features, the reported improvements seen in this retrospective review cannot be attributed to any specific component of the initiative. Nevertheless, the author speculatea that low tidal volume adherence may be one of multiple factors that impacted on overall improved outcome measures. Additionally, quarterly reporting to each center may have indirectly impacted on both process and outcome measures as these reports provide longitudinal feedback that reinforce the quality improvement culture and attitudes of participants.

Because the quarterly data reports used for this study were provided in a binary format of percent compliant, this did not permit analysis in this study of different cutoff points. Additionally, the binary format does not permit analysis of the range or the absolute change in tidal volume; therefore, the magnitude of the change was not directly examined. Also the cutoff points for compliance chosen by the database do not correspond precisely to the benchmark targets recently recommended by the ARDSnet and SCCM. However, despite all of these limitations, the data provide a description of altered practice patterns that demonstrates a positive improvement over the implementation timeline.

The author encountered considerable practice variation at baseline among participating centers for all process and outcome measures. For example, baseline VDR ranged from 0.66 up to 1.90. This underlying variability in practice pattern despite robust recommendations for best practice and published guidelines demonstrates the scope of the problem and points to the significant challenges faced by TeleICU providers in a community-based setting. The lack of uniformity and resulting large standard error may limit the detection of cross-sectional differences.

In addition to these hospital-based challenges, a *reporting rule change* in Q4 2011 for APACHE IV altered the definition of ventilator day as any part of a calendar day as well as to include patients receiving noninvasive positive pressure ventilation. Thus, these extended inclusion criteria changed by the central database may have attenuated the magnitude of VDR reduction in the most recent quarter. This diminished effect would occur because of inclusion of more patients, and longer duration would generate a larger numerator in VDR calculation.

Moreover, one subscribing hospital included in cross-sectional analysis (Hospital 1) declined to adopt structured ventilator rounds, though they continued to receive quarterly data and feedback on performance during the follow-up interval. This center's lack of improvement compared with all other centers suggests that, in the absence of daily ventilator rounds, neither preimplementation meetings nor quarterly feedback were sufficient to lead to measurable outcome differences.

In conclusion, variable practices among ICUs pose challenges to TeleICU-led process improvement. Despite this, the implementation of TeleICU-directed ventilator rounds was associated with improved and durable adherence to LPV strategies and significant reductions in the VDR and ICU mortality ratio. These data support the hypothesis that this process improvement effort contributed to the observed changes.

Key Points: Best Practice Guidelines for Telemedicine Intensive Care Unit–Directed Performance Improvement: Data/Resources/Team-Building Essentials

1. Good data strategies
   a. Remember the aphorism *you can't improve what you can't measure*
   b. Use automated data-entry systems whenever possible
   c. Enhance the delta; use benchmarked data and incorporate APACHE IV–predicted values to demonstrate performance relative to standards
   d. Consider utilizing specialized statistical tools such as control chart analysis to enhance data the capacity to detect special cause effect
2. Resource strategies
   a. Regard the TeleICU service as a source of manpower and data acquisition that can bolster the capability of the bedside team
   b. Combine the task of PI with routine clinical monitoring and management activities whenever possible

3. Team-building essentials
   a. Emphasize the shared responsibility and shared goals across the TeleICU/bedside services to enhance a culture of safety
   b. Strategically empower all members of the multidisciplinary team to have an essential role in all facets of the PI tasks, from planning, implementation, and sharing of results
   c. Make the process reiterative and share in the successes as well as combining efforts to troubleshoot

REFERENCES

1. Curtis JR, Cook DJ, Wall RJ, et al. Intensive care unit quality improvement: a "how-to" guide for the interdisciplinary team. Crit Care Med 2006;34:211–8.
2. Yang M, Fry MJ, Raikhelkar J, et al. A model to create an efficient and equitable admission policy for patients arriving to the cardiothoracic ICU. Crit Care Med 2013;41(2):414–22.
3. Reader TW, Flin R, Mearns K, et al. Developing a team performance framework for the intensive care unit. Crit Care Med 2009;37:1787–93.
4. Lilly CM, Shawn C, Zhao H, et al. Hospital mortality, length of stay, and preventable complications among critically ill patients before and after tele-ICU reengineering of critical care processes. JAMA 2011;305(21):2175–83.
5. Young LB, Chan PS, Lu X, et al. Impact of telemedicine intensive care unit coverage on patient outcomes. Arch Intern Med 2011;171(6):498–506.
6. Willmitch B, Goembeski S, Sandy SS, et al. Clinical outcomes after telemedicine intensive care unit implementation. Crit Care Med 2012;40(2):450–4.
7. Mohammed MA, Worthington P, Woodhall WH. Plotting basic control charts: tutorial notes for healthcare practitioners. Qual Saf Health Care 2008;17: 137–45.
8. Wilcox ME, Wiener-Kronish JP. Telemedicine in the intensive care unit: effect of a remote intensivist on outcomes. JAMA Intern Med 2014;174(7):1167–9.
9. Thomas EJ, Lucke JF, Wueste L, et al. Association of telemedicine for remote monitoring of intensive care patients with mortality, complications and length of stay. JAMA 2009;302(24):2671–8.
10. Morrison JL, Cai Q, Davis N, et al. Clinical and economic outcomes of the electronic intensive care unit: results from two community hospitals. Crit Care Med 2010;38(1):2–8.
11. Young LB, Chan PS, Cram P. Staff acceptance of Tele-ICU coverage: a systematic review. Chest 2011;139:279–88.
12. Kalb T, Raikhelkar J, Meyer S, et al. A multicenter population-based effectiveness study of teleintensive care unit-directed ventilator rounds demonstrating improved adherence to a protective lung strategy, decreased ventilator duration, and decreased intensive care unit mortality. J Crit Care 2014. http://dx.doi.org/10.1016/j.jcrc.2014.02.017 [pii:S0883–9441(14)00073-2].
13. Kalhan R, Mikkelsen M, Dedhiya P, et al. Underuse of lung protective ventilation: analysis of potential factors to explain physician behavior. Crit Care Med 2006; 34(2):300–6.
14. Walkey AJ, Weiner BS. Risk factors for underuse of lung-protective ventilation in acute lung injury. J Crit Care 2012;27(3):323.
15. Wolthuis EK, Veelo DP, Choi G, et al. Mechanical ventilation with lower tidal volumes does not influence the prescription of opioids or sedatives. Crit Care 2007;11:R77.

16. Young MP, Manning HL, Wilson DL, et al. Ventilation of patients with acute lung injury and acute respiratory distress syndrome: has new evidence changed clinical practice? Crit Care Med 2004;32(6):1260–5.
17. Cooke CR, Watkins TR, Kahn JM, et al. The effect of an intensive care unit staffing model on tidal volume in patients with acute lung injury. Crit Care 2008;12:R134.
18. Mendez MP, Lazar MH, DiGiovine B, et al. Dedicated multidisciplinary ventilator bundle team and compliance with sedation vacation. Am J Crit Care 2013;22(1): 54–60.
19. Wolthuis EK, Keseioglu J, Hassink LH, et al. Adoption of lower tidal volume ventilation improves with feedback and education. Respir Care 2007;52(12):1761–6.

The Role of Telemedicine in Pediatric Critical Care

Miles S. Ellenby, MD, MS[a],*, James P. Marcin, MD, MPH[b]

KEYWORDS

- Telemedicine • Telehealth • Tele-ICU • Remote monitoring • Pediatric critical care

KEY POINTS

- Telehealth technologies can address disparities in access to care, allowing critical care providers an immediate presence at the bedside of critically ill children in remote locations.
- Telehealth technologies can improve remote diagnostic, therapeutic, and transport decisions among children receiving care in nonpediatric referral centers.
- The use of telehealth technologies has been shown to positively affect the quality and cost-effectiveness of care in intensive care units.
- The use of telehealth technologies has the potential to improve the efficiency of pediatric critical care workflows and help address shortages in workforce.

In the past 2 decades, 2 major health system factors have been identified that maximize the chances of high care quality and minimizes risks of mistakes and complications in the intensive care unit (ICU). The first factor is the regionalization of specialty ICU services. ICU regionalization is a means of concentrating medical expertise and increasing patient volumes at designated referral and tertiary care hospitals. Higher patient volumes often result in increased care efficiency and improved patient outcomes. Well-known examples include the regionalization of trauma, specialty surgical procedures, adult critical care, as well as neonatal and pediatric intensive care.[1–7]

The second factor shown to improve outcomes and quality of care in the ICU is to ensure that all patients are actively cared for by critical care physicians. In both adult and pediatric critical care medicine research, it has been shown that critically ill

Disclosures: None.
[a] Division of Critical Care Medicine, Department of Pediatrics and Anesthesiology, Telemedicine Program, Doernbecher Children's Hospital, Oregon Health & Science University, 707 Southwest Gaines Road, Mail Code CDRC-P, Portland, OR 97239-2901, USA; [b] Department of Pediatrics, University of California Davis Children's Hospital, 2516 Stockton Boulevard, Sacramento, CA 95811, USA
* Corresponding author. Division of Critical Care Medicine, Department of Pediatrics & Anesthesiology, Telemedicine Program, Doernbecher Children's Hospital, Oregon Health & Science University, 707 Southwest Gaines Road, Mail Code CDRC-P, Portland, OR 97239-2901.
E-mail address: ellenbym@ohsu.edu

patients have a lower risk of death and shorter ICU and hospital lengths of stay, and receive higher care quality when critical care physicians are involved in their management.[8–11] Researchers estimate that ICU mortality is reduced by 10% to 25% when critical care physicians direct patient care compared with ICUs where critical care physicians have little to no involvement in patient care.[8,9,12]

Despite the clear motivation that all critically ill children receive treatment in a regionalized pediatric ICU and by pediatric critical care physicians, many are cared for in less ideal settings. This finding is explained in part by simple geography, pediatric population density, and economic factors, namely the infeasibility of all hospitals to maintain the equipment and personnel to treat specific pediatric conditions.[13] The regionalization of pediatric ICUs, although increasing quality and efficiencies of care, also by its design creates disparities in access. Critically ill children from nonurban areas are frequently cared for, by necessity, in hospitals that lack the full spectrum of pediatric ICU services and/or pediatric critical care expertise.[14–16] Magnifying the problem of geography is the continued shortage of critical care physicians, both adult and pediatric, which is expected to worsen in future years.[17–19] The distribution of pediatric ICUs in the United States has been reported in the past decade.[20,21] These reports identified growing numbers of pediatric ICUs and beds as well as increased rates of baseline and 24-hour-per-day staffing by pediatric critical care physicians. The number of beds per pediatric population is similar across each US census region (national average of 1 bed per 18,542 children), although disparities still exist state by state (ranging from >1 bed per 15,000 children to <1 bed per 75,000 children). In addition, although smaller units (1–6 beds) had higher physician and nursing staffing ratios, they had lesser capacities compared with larger units to provide advanced therapies such as renal replacement and inhaled nitric oxide. Combined, regionalization and physician shortages sometimes make it difficult to guarantee that all critically ill children are treated in a timely manner, by qualified physicians, and in an appropriate full-service pediatric ICU.

Telemedicine, the interactive delivery of health care over distance using advances in telecommunication technology (ie, videoconferencing equipment), is an evolving model for care delivery that increases access, improves outcomes, and reduces costs. By improving access, both geographically and temporally, telemedicine is a potentially transformative use of technology, allowing earlier involvement of specialists in acute, life-threatening situations, as well as for many other in-person health interactions that, although not urgent, are not happening efficiently, because they are impeded by the current delivery system.[22,23] Grundy and colleagues[24] first reported on the use of telemedicine in intensive care in 1977. Access to medically underserved areas, both rural and urban, is improved by enabling critical care physicians' participation in the care of the most critically ill patients in remote locations[25,26] with the potential for cost savings primarily from reducing unnecessary patient transports, although the ultimate economic impact of telemedicine needs further study.[27,28]

By importing specialty expertise using telemedicine, emergency departments (EDs), inpatient wards, and nonspecialty ICUs are given the means to increase their capacity to provide higher quality of care to pediatric patients.[29] Critical care physicians can also increase their efficiency with these technologies so that their expertise can be disseminated to more patients at more than one ICU or hospital at a time. The use of telemedicine technologies can also reduce the need to transfer children who are less ill to referral centers, reserving the limited pediatric ICU beds for those most in need of a regionalized center.[30,31] For these reasons, the use of telemedicine by hospitals and physicians providing critical care services will continue to increase and be individualized to best fit the needs of their patients.

Although the use of telemedicine technologies can help providers of critical care services to address disparities in access to care, improve quality of care, and reduce overall health care costs, it will never replace bedside pediatric critical care physicians or eliminate the need to transfer critically ill children to regional pediatric ICUs. Instead, pediatric critical care physicians can use telemedicine and telehealth technologies as tools to assist in the remote monitoring and treatment of patients in situations where their services may not otherwise be immediately available. This article reviews how telemedicine can be used by pediatric critical care physicians and pediatric ICUs, focusing particularly on the delivery of care in remote hospital EDs, in critical care transport, in remote hospital inpatient wards, and in remote ICUs where pediatric critical care specialists are not immediately available. In addition, the role of telemedicine in neonatal intensive care is also reviewed.

TELEMEDICINE FOR CRITICALLY ILL CHILDREN IN REMOTE SETTINGS

It is well documented that critically ill children presenting to EDs without pediatric expertise receive poorer quality of care compared with the care provided in EDs with that expertise.[32–36] Many of these EDs are at times inadequately equipped to care for pediatric emergencies.[32,33,37–40] In addition, the staff working in smaller, general EDs, including physicians, nurses, pharmacists, and support staff, are often less experienced in caring for critically ill children and may do so infrequently. The combined inherent stresses of caring for a critically ill child with this lack of equipment, infrastructure, and experienced personnel results in delayed or incorrect diagnoses, suboptimal therapies, and imperfect medical management.[10,34,41,42] As a consequence, acutely ill or injured children receive a lower quality of care than children presenting to EDs in regionalized children's hospitals.[34,43–46] This is succinctly reflected in the aphorism that children are not just little adults.

The use of telemedicine technologies for disaster victims[47] or in remote or underserved EDs can be a means of obtaining subspecialty expert consultation.[48–54] Telemedicine has also been shown to be a feasible method of providing specialty expertise from the United States internationally, namely to augment the care of children with congenital heart disease in Columbia.[55] The benefit of using this technology as opposed to using the telephone (the current standard of care) is that the consultant (ie, the pediatric critical care physician) has the ability to have a virtual presence at the patient's bedside. The consultant has full control of the remote camera, including movement about the room and high-resolution zoom, allowing access to high-definition video views of the patient, the treating providers, the family, as well as monitors and other medical equipment (**Fig. 1**). Previous studies have shown that the use of telemedicine in the ED to deliver consultations is similar to in-person consultations in terms of diagnostic accuracy, treatment plans, and plans for disposition.[29,49,56–59] The use of telemedicine to urgently obtain a consultation from a neurologist in the ED to treat a patient with an acute stroke is now common practice.[58–61] Similarly, telemedicine is used to provide emergency medicine consultations to critical access hospitals, which are staffed by physician assistants.[62] Both of these examples have been shown to result in high-quality, cost-effective care.[62–64]

There is increasing evidence and acceptance that providing pediatric critical care consultations to remote EDs for critically ill children can improve the quality of care and increase provider, patient, and parent/guardian satisfaction.[57,65] Three studies have describe how pediatric critical care physicians use telemedicine to provide consultations to critically ill children presenting to several rural EDs.[29,57,65] Heath

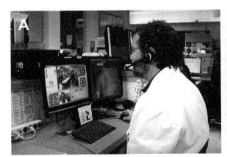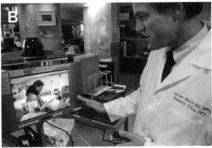

Fig. 1. The authors delivering pediatric critical care consults.

and colleagues[57] at the University of Vermont concluded that use of telemedicine was associated with improved patient care and was superior to telephone consultations.[66] A study by Dharmar and colleagues[67] showed that patients receiving telemedicine consultations in remote EDs received higher overall care quality compared with similar patients receiving telephone consultations.[65] Both of these programs also reported that referring ED physicians more frequently changed their diagnoses and/or therapeutic interventions than when consultations were provided by telephone. In addition, the use of telemedicine to provide critical care consultations has also been shown to result in significantly higher parent/guardian satisfaction and perceived quality compared with telephone consultations.[65]

A recent survey of programs providing pediatric critical care consults to EDs identified 9 active, 5 planned, and 3 closed programs in the United States (**Table 1**).[68] Success factors for these programs included identifying spoke hospitals based on receptivity and cultivating clinical champions at the spoke facilities. Several barriers

Table 1
Current programs

Program	Years in Operation	Lead Department at Hub Site	Number of Spoke Sites	Estimated Consults Per Year
University of California, Davis	2003–present	ED	18	48
Boston Children's Hospital	2012	Pediatric ICU	1	a
Vermont Children's Hospital at Fletcher Allen Health Care	2003–present	Pediatric ICU	12	12
University of Arkansas	2007–present	ED	24+	Not reported
Oregon Health and Science University	2007–present	Pediatric ICU	10	85
University of New Mexico	2012–present	ED	1	a
Massachusetts General	1998	Pediatric ICU	30	40
Eastern Maine Medical Center	2005	Pediatric ICU and trauma surgery	15	40
Children's Hospital of Orange County	2007	Pediatric ICU	2	50

[a] Missing for programs less than 1 year old at the time of the survey.

Adapted from Uscher-Pines L, Kahn JM. Barriers and facilitators to pediatric emergency telemedicine in the United States. Telemed J E Health 2014;20(11):990–6.

were also identified, including credentialing, workflow integration at both sites because telemedicine consults require more time compared to telephone consults, usability of the technology, lack of physician buy-in, and misaligned incentives between the sites. Uneven reimbursement was also mentioned but was not perceived as a major issue because many programs operate independently of reimbursement. Note that most of the hub sites are academic institutions that may have motivations other than reimbursement.

Overall, although more research is needed, there is mounting evidence that pediatric critical care consultations to rural and underserved EDs using telemedicine can be used to help address disparities in access to specialists and, in doing so, improve the overall quality of care. It is also likely, that because of better care and the reduction in unnecessary transports, telemedicine consultations to rural and underserved EDs can be provided in a cost-efficient manner that reduces the health care costs that would otherwise be incurred if telemedicine were not used.[69]

TELEMEDICINE DURING TRANSPORT OF CRITICALLY ILL PEDIATRIC PATIENTS

The use of telemedicine by physicians to assist in the care of critically ill patients during transport could have the potential to improve processes of care at several levels. For example, telemedicine could allow physicians to be an immediate part of the monitoring, identification, and management of changes in the patient's status that occur during transport. With more immediate physician supervision using telemedicine, medical decisions, including new medication orders, have the potential to occur more rapidly and efficiently than without direct physician supervision.

At present, mobile telephone technologies are used to transmit 2-way audio as well as data, including electrocardiogram data. However, to create a model of care that uses telemedicine during transport, much more robust mobile broadband telecommunications are needed. Only a few transport programs in the United States use these technologies because high-quality broadband mobile telecommunication is expensive and not always or easily available,[70] particularly if continuous video transmission or large amounts of data streaming is desired. Common methods of transmitting video include the use of high-fidelity cell-phone services (sometimes combining several cell-phone lines) and the use of the Internet, which can be available with citywide Wi-Fi or satellite services.[71,72] Although satellite technologies can be used to provide mobile telemedicine connections, this technology is most often prohibitively expensive.

There have been anecdotal reports documenting the feasibility of cell-phone and Wi-Fi transmitted telemedicine consultations during transport. In one study, the outcomes of adult patients with simulated trauma were compared among scenarios that used telemedicine and scenarios that used telephone communications during transport.[73] Use of telemedicine resulted in a reduction in adverse clinical events, including fewer episodes of desaturation and hypotension, and less tachycardia compared with identical simulated patients without telemedicine use. In addition, recognition rates for key physiologic signs and the need for critical interventions were higher in the transport simulations that used telemedicine.[73]

These data are encouraging and support the possibility that telemedicine can be used during patient transport. However, until more reliable and affordable mobile telecommunications are available to implement telemedicine during transport and until more research is conducted on the impact that telemedicine has during transport and on workflow, the effectiveness and benefit of this technology remain undetermined.

CRITICAL CARE TELEMEDICINE CONSULTATIONS FOR HOSPITALIZED CHILDREN

Pediatric critical care services are more regionalized and fewer than adult critical care services. Therefore children living in nonurban communities who may need critical care services are often transported to a pediatric ICU, exposing them to the inherent risks and costs. At times, pediatric patients who are not critically ill are overtriaged and transferred to the regional center, because there may be a need for the specialty services provided by the pediatric ICU.[74] Adding to this inefficiency, regionalized quaternary pediatric ICUs frequently run at full capacity. The transfer of some pediatric patients to a quaternary pediatric referral center is often not necessary if there is a closer hospital with adequate pediatric capabilities, such as a level II or community pediatric ICU, an intermediate or step-down pediatric care unit, or a general ICU with pediatric expertise.[75]

Admitting some of the less ill children to hospitals other than regional, quaternary referral centers can result in high quality of care provided with shorter length of stays, less resource use, and lower costs.[76–78] It is therefore logical that some mildly or moderately ill children (eg, children with asthma who require continuous albuterol or children with known diabetes and mild diabetic ketoacidosis) can be cared for in level II or community pediatric ICUs or other nonchildren's hospital ICUs under the care of pediatric nurses and physicians with supervision from a regional children's hospital pediatric critical care team using telemedicine and remote monitoring.[29]

Telemedicine can be used by pediatric critical care clinicians using a broad range of applications to assist in the care of hospitalized children in a variety of clinical scenarios.[79] Physician consultations, nurse and physician monitoring, and medical oversight can range from a simple model of intermittent, need-based consultations (reactive model) to a model that integrates continuous oversight via monitoring and proactive medical decision making (continuous model).[80] In a reactive model, a pediatric critical care physician can provide bedside telemedicine consultations to patients in remote EDs, inpatient wards, high-acuity units, or ICUs. Such consultations could prompt a variety of clinical interventions, including recommendations on diagnostic studies, medications, or other therapies. The consultation may also conclude the need to transport the patient to the regional pediatric ICU. This type of model could result in a range of interventions from a 1-time consultation to multiple videoconferencing interactions during the course of the day or hospital stay.[25,81]

In the continuous model, oversight by critical care physicians and nurses is provided by telemedicine in combination with comprehensive electronic remote monitoring. In such a model, a remote team of physicians and nurses is able to monitor many patient beds, often covering several ICUs. This continuous oversight model of telemedicine is more proactive with medical interventions and often involves nontelemedicine guidelines such as the implementation of evidence-based protocols. This electronic ICU is created by centralizing electronic health records, ICU monitoring technologies, and nurse/physician video oversight. Tele-ICUs can be created internally by large health systems, or can be contracted out to third party technology and physician organizations that specialize in remote ICU monitoring services.

Reactive Model

A pediatric critical care telemedicine program based on the consultative model has been successfully used in caring for mildly to moderately ill children in remote ICUs by several programs.[25,82] One such model could involve pediatric critical care physicians from a regional pediatric ICU connecting to the bedside for consultations to a referring neonatologist, general pediatrician, adult critical care physician, and/or surgeon caring for an infant, child, or adolescent in a community or combined pediatric-adult ICU. The bedside nurse or physician could initiate a request for consultation either from the regional pediatric critical care nurse or physician. Such a model would also require compliance with critical care best practices and maintenance of pediatric critical care training, advanced life support certifications, and participation in quality assurance programs.[25,81]

In this model of care, telemedicine consultations from pediatric critical care physicians should be available 24 hours per day, 7 days per week. Consultations should consist of a full history (with referring physician, nurse, and/or parent/guardian) and a physical examination, which may require the use of telemedicine peripheral devices (such as a stethoscope, otoscope, ophthalmoscope, and/or a general examination camera) or reported physical findings from bedside clinical staff. The consultation should include review of pertinent radiographs, medical records, and laboratories. Radiographs are often made available via electronic file sharing. Follow-up consultations can be conducted at the discretion of the consulting critical care physician or as requested by the referring physician or bedside nurse. At any time after the initial or follow-up consultation, the patient can be transported to the regional pediatric ICU based on specialty needs of the patient, the discretion of the referring or consulting physicians with considerations to nurse and physician comfort, and/or parental preference.

Published data from a consultative telemedicine program show excellent clinical outcomes, including mortality and length of stay, similar to severity-adjusted benchmark data from a set of national pediatric ICUs.[25,81] This program has reported a high degree of satisfaction among remote providers and parents/guardians, and allowed patients to remain in their local communities, thereby lessening the burden on family members. In addition, implementation of this consultative telemedicine model resulted in an overall reduction in health care costs because of more appropriate transport use and decreased use of the more costly regional pediatric ICU.[69] Moreover, the use of telemedicine to assist with cardiopulmonary resuscitation has been reported.[83]

There is a trend within pediatric critical care toward 24-hour in-house attending-level coverage, but many pediatric ICUs continue to use a system of overnight coverage by trainees at the bedside, with attending backup from home. Another novel use of telemedicine allows at-home pediatric ICU physicians to connect to the ICU at night to assist the on-site team in a reactive mode.[84] This method has been shown to be feasible, although it has not been rigorously assessed with regard to quality. The reactive telemedicine model has also been reported by other pediatric specialists to provide inpatient consultations, including cardiology consultations and ethics consultations.[85,86]

The neonatal ICU (NICU) has also been a venue for telemedicine, using several different models to influence the care of newborns as well as improve the triage of high-risk obstetric patients so that they may deliver in the best location for immediate care of the potentially critically ill neonate. Hall and colleagues[87] in Arkansas established a statewide system for high-risk obstetrics and neonatology: the Antenatal and Neonatal Guidelines, Education, and Learning System (ANGELS). This multifaceted program includes both obstetric and neonatal remote rounding, consultation, and education. The institution of the network has resulted in decreased deliveries of very low birth weight neonates in hospitals without NICUs and was associated with decreased statewide infant mortality.[88] Similar to other multipronged systematic interventions in health care, it is unclear which aspect provided the most benefit. With respect to neonatal specialty consultation, telemedicine has also been used to provide remote evaluations for surgical conditions[89] and genetic and neurologic disorders.[90] Tele-echocardiography has been used with both a store-and-forward methodology as well as by a real-time consultation with a pediatric cardiologist. A recent multicenter study investigated the impact of telemedicine on the care of newborns with suspected congenital heart disease.[91] Data were analyzed on matched pairs of neonates with mild or no heart disease and showed shorter time to diagnosis and significantly decreased need for transport, length of hospitalization, and ICU stay in the telemedicine cohort compared with the control group. In addition, the use of indomethacin to close a patent ductus arteriosus and the use of inotropic support was less in the telemedicine group, thereby showing that telemedicine is both diagnostic and can reduce exposure to risky, unnecessary treatments and transports. Researchers in Australia studied the costs of implementation and potential savings from a neonatal telemedicine program.[92] Over the course of 12 months, 19 telemedicine consultations resulted in 5 avoided transports, resulting in cost savings even when accounting for the cost of implementation.

Continuous Oversight Model

When telemedicine is integrated with continuous remote electronic monitoring and integration of electronic health records, the result is a telepresence ICU system. This system is a more comprehensive and proactive care model that involves around-the-clock monitoring by critical care nurses and physicians. In this model of care, the role of the critical care specialist can range from involvement only during patient emergencies to more active involvement, including ongoing communication with remote providers directing changes in care and therapies. Using this continuous oversight model, initial research studies comparing preintervention with postintervention outcomes suggested a non–statistically significant reduction in severity-adjusted ICU mortality, severity-adjusted hospital mortality, and incidence of some ICU complications, and decreased ICU length of stay.[93,94] However, the studies found no significant reduction in overall hospital length of stay and were conducted by teams of investigators affiliated with the proprietary remote ICU telemedicine company used in the investigations.

There have been several subsequent studies evaluating the impact of the continuous remote oversight ICU model in a variety of adult ICU settings. In a large study conducted at 6 ICUs in a large US health care system, a similar preintervention versus postintervention study found that implementation of an integrated telemedicine and remote monitoring program did not have a large impact on evaluated care.[95] This study reported no difference in ICU mortality, hospital mortality, ICU length of stay, or hospital length of stay. However, the researchers found that, among the subset of patients with higher involvement of remote telemedicine providers, outcomes, including survival, were improved.[95] Using the data from this study, another group of investigators researched the costs and cost-effectiveness of the tele-ICU program.[96] Daily average ICU and hospital costs after the implementation of the program increased by 28% and 34%, respectively. The investigators concluded that the cost-effectiveness of the continuous oversight program was limited to the most severely ill patients.[96] Another recent study undertaken in 7 hospitals within the US Department of Veteran Affairs system found no evidence for reduced mortality or length of stay with the use of telemedicine.[97] However, the investigators point to limitations, including unequal adoption across the sites and an extremely low baseline mortality in both groups, suggesting a lower acuity population.

Several more recent studies in smaller hospital settings found conflicting results.[98–100] In one report in which the tele-ICU was used to monitor 4 ICUs in 2 community hospitals, investigators found no reduction in ICU mortality, hospital mortality,

ICU length of stay, or hospital length of stay.[100] In the same year, in a similarly designed study of a single academic community hospital, the continuous remote oversight ICU telemedicine model resulted in a statistically significant reduction in mortality from 21.4% at baseline to 14.7%. These investigators also found a significant reduction in ICU length of stay from 4.06 days at baseline to 3.77 days, which remained significant even after adjustment for case mix and severity of illness.[99]

Researchers from the University of Massachusetts Memorial Critical Care Operations Group evaluated 7 adult ICUs on 2 campuses of a single academic medical center where a similar continuous oversight telemedicine program was implemented. These researchers found that the tele-ICU program was associated with significant improvements in several clinical outcomes.[101] The adherence to critical care best practices, including guidelines for prevention of deep vein thrombosis, stress ulcers, ventilator-associated pneumonia, catheter-related bloodstream infections, and guidelines for cardiovascular protection, all significantly improved. In addition, there was a relative reduction in unadjusted and risk-adjusted ICU mortality by 13% and 20%, respectively. Further, both risk-adjusted hospital mortality ICU and hospital length of stay were significantly decreased.[101,102] More recently, these investigators evaluated the impact of the tele-ICU model in a multicenter study across 56 ICUs in 32 hospitals, resulting in a sample of 118,990 patients (107,432 in the telemedicine group and 11,558 controls).[103] The implementation of the ICU telemedicine program again showed a statistically significant decrease in mortality, as well as lengths of stay, in both the ICU and hospital settings. They also identified 6 individual ICU processes that were associated with an improvement in at least 1 of the 4 major outcomes, namely earlier intensivist management; coordinated, timely usage of performance information; achievement of higher rates of adherence to best practices; shorter alarm response times; more frequent interdisciplinary rounds; and a more effective ICU committee.[103]

There have been at least 2 meta-analyses that have combined published data evaluating ICU telemedicine's impact on patient outcomes. In one, researchers found that, among 13 eligible studies involving 35 ICUs, there was a significant reduction in ICU mortality (pooled odds ratio, 0.80), but no impact on in-hospital mortality for patients admitted to the ICU.[104] Remote ICU telemedicine coverage was also associated with a reduction in ICU length of stay by 1.3 days, but there was no statistically significant reduction in hospital length of stay.[104] In another, researchers reviewed 11 eligible studies and the continuous remote oversight telemedicine model resulted in statistically significant reductions in ICU and hospital mortality (pooled risk ratio, 0.79 and 0.89, respectively) as well as ICU and hospital lengths of stay.[105] All studies included in both of these meta-analyses were combined assessments that compared pretelemedicine outcomes with post-telemedicine outcomes, which are subject to significant bias. As shown by the inconsistent conclusions that were reached by 2 different meta-analyses that analyzed virtually identical data, there is a need to conduct more rigorous studies in which timelines are concurrent and/or patients and ICUs are randomized as part of a larger trial.[106,107] Given the unclear efficacy of the tele-ICU model, researchers undertook a systematic review and analysis of the literature with regard to the costs associated with implementation.[108] They further obtained the costs within a network of 7 US Department of Veteran Affairs hospitals. The literature suggested a combined implementation and first-year operation costs in the range of $50,000 to $100,000 per monitored ICU bed. Similar costs were identified within the Veterans Affairs hospitals.

The reasons why some continuous oversight telemedicine programs have resulted in significantly improved outcomes whereas others have not is likely multifactorial and related to how the programs were implemented and supported. In general, if ICUs experienced improvements in clinical outcomes, the centralized, monitoring critical care teams seemed to work more proactively and were involved in care of a greater proportion of patients. In contrast, in ICUs that did not experience improvements in clinical outcomes, the ICUs often limited the participation of the centralized, monitoring critical care teams. In addition, some studies that did not find improvements in clinical outcomes often did not simultaneously implement clinical improvement programs so the degree of benefit seems to be related to the extent to which the telemedicine, remote monitoring, and collaboration between the monitoring and monitored teams are mutually embraced and whether the program is supported as a means of creating sustainable improvements in ICU care.[101,109,110] These issues were further explored in a qualitative study using semistructured interviews and site observations within a US Department of Veteran Affairs tele-ICU network.[111] The investigators concluded that the implementation process is complex and disruptive to previous workflows and cultures of practice. Acceptance was complicated by inconsistent knowledge about the system and an investment in educating and training of ICU staff is likely to lead to greater adoption and potentially greater efficacy.

THE FUTURE OF TELEMEDICINE IN PEDIATRIC INTENSIVE CARE UNITS

In conclusion, the utility of a care model that uses telemedicine to assist in the treatment of infants and children hospitalized in remote hospitals or ICUs is promising, but remains controversial because of a lack of evidence. It is known that telemedicine technology, in and of itself, does not result in improved care. Telemedicine is a technological tool that can enable providers to provide better care. Telemedicine needs to be thoughtfully integrated into partnering institutions in a well-defined and collaborative effort, and in these cases it can result in improvements in access and quality for mildly or moderately ill children.[112-114] Similar to other quality improvement efforts, for the success of a telemedicine partnership, there must be firm support from administrators, physicians, nurses, and other clinical providers on both sides of telemedicine.

It is likely that the use of telemedicine in pediatric critical care and in pediatric ICUs will increase. Telehealth technologies can allow specialists, including pediatric critical care physicians, to extend their expertise more quickly and easily to locations in need of their services by eliminating the time and geographic barriers to access. The potential advantages are numerous, and include improved access, improved efficiencies, improved quality, and more cost-effective care. All of these work to the advantage of patients, patients' families, remote clinicians, and regional health care systems.

In addition, as telemedicine connections between remote hospitals and regionalized pediatric ICUs are enhanced, pediatric critical care physicians can better educate remote providers in the care of critically ill children. Telemedicine technologies will become more integrated into the practice of medicine, similarly to computerized physician order entry and the electronic health record. Different models of care require different technologies depending on the needs of the patients, the remote hospitals, and the regional pediatric ICUs. More data will help clinicians determine where, when, and for whom the telemedicine technologies are most clinically and economically effective.[114]

REFERENCES

1. Birkmeyer JD, Finlayson EV, Birkmeyer CM. Volume standards for high-risk surgical procedures: potential benefits of the leapfrog initiative. Surgery 2001; 130(3):415–22.

2. Phibbs CS, Bronstein JM, Buxton E, et al. The effects of patient volume and level of care at the hospital of birth on neonatal mortality. JAMA 1996;276(13):1054–9.

3. Tilford JM, Simpson PM, Green JW, et al. Volume-outcome relationships in pediatric intensive care units. Pediatrics 2000;106(2):289.

4. Marcin JP, Li Z, Kravitz RL, et al. The CABG surgery volume–outcome relationship: temporal trends and selection effects in California, 1998–2004. Health Serv Res 2008;43(1):174–92.

5. Marcin JP, Song J, Leigh JP. The impact of pediatric intensive care unit volume on mortality: a hierarchical instrumental variable analysis. Pediatr Crit Care Med 2005;6(2):136–41.

6. Finks JF, Osborne NH, Birkmeyer JD. Trends in hospital volume and operative mortality for high-risk surgery. N Engl J Med 2011;364(22):2128–37.

7. Lorch SA, Myers S, Carr B. The regionalization of pediatric health care. Pediatrics 2010;126(6):1182–90.

8. Pronovost PJ, Angus DC, Dorman T, et al. Physician staffing patterns and clinical outcomes in critically ill patients: a systematic review. JAMA 2002;288:2151–62.

9. Blunt MC, Burchett KR. Out-of-hours consultant cover and case-mix-adjusted mortality in intensive care. Lancet 2000;356:735–6.

10. Pollack MM, Alexander SR, Clarke N, et al. Improved outcomes from tertiary center pediatric intensive care: a statewide comparison of tertiary and nontertiary care facilities. Crit Care Med 1991;19:150–9.

11. Pollack MM, Cuerdon TT, Patel KM, et al. Impact of quality-of-care factors on pediatric intensive care unit mortality. JAMA 1994;272:941–96.

12. Wallace DJ, Angus DC, Barnato AE, et al. Nighttime intensivist staffing and mortality among critically ill patients. N Engl J Med 2012;366:2093–101.

13. Menke TJ, Wray NP. When does regionalization of expensive medical care save money? Health Serv Manage Res 2001;14(2):116–24.

14. Odetola FO, Miller WC, Davis MM, et al. The relationship between the location of pediatric intensive care unit facilities and child death from trauma: a county-level ecologic study. J Pediatr 2005;147:74–7.

15. Kanter RK. Regional variation in child mortality at hospitals lacking a pediatric intensive care unit. Crit Care Med 2002;30:94–9.

16. Austin JD. Critically ill children in non-paediatric intensive care units: a survey, review and proposal for practice. Anaesth Intensive Care 2007;35(6):961–7.

17. Angus DC, Kelley MA, Schmitz RJ, et al. Caring for the critically ill patient. Current and projected workforce requirements for care of the critically ill and patients with pulmonary disease: can we meet the requirements of an aging population? JAMA 2000;284:2762–70.

18. American Academy of Pediatrics Committee on Pediatric Workforce. Pediatrician workforce statement. Pediatrics 2005;116:263–9.

19. Kelley MA, Angus D, Chalfin DB, et al. The critical care crisis in the United States: a report from the profession. Chest 2004;125:1514–7.

20. Randolph AG, Gonzales CA, Cortellini L, et al. Growth of pediatric intensive care units in the United States from 1995 to 2001. J Pediatr 2004;144(6):792–8.

21. Odetola FO, Clark SJ, Freed GL, et al. A national survey of pediatric critical care resources in the United States. Pediatrics 2005;115(4):e382–6.

22. Kvedar J, Coye MJ, Everett W. Connected health: a review of technologies and strategies to improve patient care with telemedicine and telehealth. Health Aff (Millwood) 2014;33(2):194–9.

23. Marcin JP, Ellis J, Mawis R, et al. Using telemedicine to provide pediatric sub-specialty care to children with special health care needs in an underserved rural community. Pediatrics 2004;113:1–6.

24. Grundy BL, Crawford P, Jones PK, et al. Telemedicine in critical care: an experiment in health care delivery. JACEP 1977;6(10):439–44.

25. Marcin JP, Nesbitt TS, Kallas HJ, et al. Use of telemedicine to provide pediatric critical care inpatient consultations to underserved rural northern California. J Pediatr 2004;144:375–80.

26. Mueller KJ, Potter AJ, MacKinney AC, et al. Lessons from tele-emergency: improving care quality and health outcomes by expanding support for rural care systems. Health Aff (Millwood) 2014;33(2):228–34.

27. Davalos ME, French MT, Burdick AE, et al. Economic evaluation of telemedicine: review of the literature and research guidelines for benefit-cost analysis. Telemed J E Health 2009;15(10):933–48.

28. Mistry H, Garnvwa H, Oppong R. Critical appraisal of published systematic reviews assessing the cost-effectiveness of telemedicine studies. Telemed J E Health 2014;20(7):1–10.

29. Labarbera JM, Ellenby MS, Bouressa P, et al. The impact of telemedicine intensivist support and a pediatric hospitalist program on a community hospital. Telemed J E Health 2013;19(10):760–6.

30. Haskins PA, Ellis DG, Mayrose J. Predicted utilization of emergency medical services telemedicine in decreasing ambulance transports. Prehosp Emerg Care 2002;6:445–8.

31. Tsai SH, Kraus J, Wu HR, et al. The effectiveness of video-telemedicine for screening of patients requesting emergency air medical transport (EAMT). J Trauma 2007;62:504–11.

32. Athey J, Dean JM, Ball J, et al. Ability of hospitals to care for pediatric emergency patients. Pediatr Emerg Care 2001;17:170–4.

33. McGillivray D, Nijssen-Jordan C, Kramer MS, et al. Critical pediatric equipment availability in Canadian hospital emergency departments. Ann Emerg Med 2001;37:371–6.

34. Dharmar M, Marcin JP, Romano PS, et al. Quality of care of children in the emergency department: association with hospital setting and physician training. J Pediatr 2008;153(6):783–9.

35. Bowman SM, Zimmerman FJ, Christakis DA, et al. Hospital characteristics associated with the management of pediatric splenic injuries. JAMA 2005;294:2611–7.

36. Li J, Monuteaux MC, Bachur RG. Interfacility transfers of noncritically ill children to academic pediatric emergency departments. Pediatrics 2012;130:83–92.

37. Middleton KR, Burt CW. Availability of pediatric services and equipment in Emergency Departments: United States, 2002–03. Adv Data 2006;(367):1–16.

38. Gausche-Hill M, Schmitz C, Lewis RJ. Pediatric preparedness of US emergency departments: a 2003 survey. Pediatrics 2007;120:1229–37.

39. Bourgeois FT, Shannon MW. Emergency care for children in pediatric and general emergency departments. Pediatr Emerg Care 2007;23:94–102.

40. Burt CW, Middleton KR. Factors associated with ability to treat pediatric emergencies in US hospitals. Pediatr Emerg Care 2007;23:681–9.

41. Tilford JM, Roberson PK, Lensing S, et al. Improvement in pediatric critical care outcomes. Crit Care Med 2000;28:601–63.

42. Keeler EB, Rubenstein LV, Kahn KL, et al. Hospital characteristics and quality of care. JAMA 1992;268:1709–14.

43. Seidel JS, Henderson DP, Ward P, et al. Pediatric prehospital care in urban and rural areas. Pediatrics 1991;88:681–90.
44. Seidel JS, Hornbein M, Yoshiyama K, et al. Emergency medical services and the pediatric patient: are the needs being met? Pediatrics 1984;73:769–72.
45. Durch JS, Lohr KN. From the Institute of Medicine. JAMA 1993;270:929.
46. Durch J, Lohr KN, Institute of Medicine (US) Committee on Pediatric Emergency Medical Services. Emergency medical services for children. Washington, DC: National Academy Press; 1993. p. xvi, 396. Available at: http://www.nap.edu/readingroom/records/0309048885.html.
47. Burke RV, Berg BM, Vee P, et al. Using robotic telecommunications to triage pediatric disaster victims. J Pediatr Surg 2012;47:221–4.
48. Lambrecht CJ. Emergency physicians' roles in a clinical telemedicine network. Ann Emerg Med 1997;30:670–4.
49. Brennan JA, Kealy JA, Gerardi LH, et al. Telemedicine in the emergency department: a randomized controlled trial. J Telemed Telecare 1999;5:18–22.
50. Brennan JA, Kealy JA, Gerardi LH, et al. A randomized controlled trial of telemedicine in an emergency department. J Telemed Telecare 1998;4:18–20.
51. Stamford P, Bickford T, Hsiao H, et al. The significance of telemedicine in a rural emergency department. IEEE Eng Med Biol Mag 1999;18:45–52.
52. Rogers FB, Ricci M, Caputo M, et al. The use of telemedicine for real-time video consultation between trauma center and community hospital in a rural setting improves early trauma care: preliminary results. J Trauma 2001;51:1037–41.
53. Latifi R, Hadeed GJ, Rhee P, et al. Initial experiences and outcomes of telepresence in the management of trauma and emergency surgical patients. Am J Surg 2009;198:905–10.
54. Hicks LL, Boles KE, Hudson ST, et al. Using telemedicine to avoid transfer of rural emergency department patients. J Rural Health 2001;17:220–8.
55. Munoz RA, Burbano NH, Motoa MV, et al. Telemedicine in pediatric cardiac critical care. Telemed J E Health 2012;18(2):132–6.
56. Kofos D, Pitetti R, Orr R, et al. Telemedicine in pediatric transport: a feasibility study. Pediatrics 1998;102:E58.
57. Heath B, Salerno R, Hopkins A, et al. Pediatric critical care telemedicine in rural underserved emergency departments. Pediatr Crit Care Med 2009;10(5):588–91.
58. Meyer BC, Raman R, Hemmen T, et al. Efficacy of site-independent telemedicine in the STRokE DOC trial: a randomised, blinded, prospective study. Lancet Neurol 2008;7:787–95.
59. Demaerschalk BM, Raman R, Ernstrom K, et al. Efficacy of telemedicine for stroke: pooled analysis of the stroke team remote evaluation using a digital observation camera (STRokE DOC) and STRokE DOC Arizona telestroke trials. Telemed J E Health 2012;18:230–7.
60. Emsley H, Blacker K, Davies P, et al. Telestroke. When location, location, location doesn't matter. Health Serv J 2010;120:24–5.
61. Pervez MA, Silva G, Masrur S, et al. Remote supervision of IV-tPA for acute ischemic stroke by telemedicine or telephone before transfer to a regional stroke center is feasible and safe. Stroke 2010;41:e18–24.
62. Galli R, Keith JC, McKenzie K, et al. TelEmergency: a novel system for delivering emergency care to rural hospitals. Ann Emerg Med 2008;51:275–84.
63. Henderson K. TelEmergency: distance emergency care in rural emergency departments using nurse practitioners. J Emerg Nurs 2006;32:388–93.
64. Nelson RE, Saltzman GM, Skalabrin EJ, et al. The cost-effectiveness of telestroke in the treatment of acute ischemic stroke. Neurology 2011;77:1590–8.

65. Dharmar MR, Romano PS, Kuppermann N, et al. Impact of pediatric telemedicine consultations on critically ill children in rural emergency departments. Crit Care Med 2013;41:2388–95.

66. Dharmar M, Marcin JP. A picture is worth a thousand words: critical care consultations to emergency departments using telemedicine. Pediatr Crit Care Med 2009;10:606–7.

67. Dharmar M, Marcin JP, Kuppermann N, et al. A new implicit review instrument for measuring quality of care delivered to pediatric patients in the emergency department. BMC Emerg Med 2007;7:13.

68. Uscher-Pines L, Kahn JM. Barriers and facilitators to pediatric emergency telemedicine in the United States. Telemed J E Health 2014;20(11):990–6.

69. Marcin JP, Nesbitt TS, Struve S, et al. Financial benefits of a pediatric intensive care unit-based telemedicine program to a rural adult intensive care unit: impact of keeping acutely ill and injured children in their local community. Telemed J E Health 2004;10:1–5.

70. Liman TG, Winter B, Waldschmidt C, et al. Telestroke ambulances in prehospital stroke management: concept and pilot feasibility study. Stroke 2012;43: 2086–90.

71. Qureshi A, Shih E, Fan I, et al. Improving patient care by unshackling telemedicine: adaptively aggregating wireless networks to facilitate continuous collaboration. AMIA Annu Symp Proc 2010;2010:662–6.

72. Hsieh JC, Lin BX, Wu FR, et al. Ambulance 12-lead electrocardiography transmission via cell phone technology to cardiologists. Telemed J E Health 2010;16: 910–5.

73. Charash WE, Caputo MP, Clark H, et al. Telemedicine to a moving ambulance improves outcome after trauma in simulated patients. J Trauma 2011;71:49–55.

74. Wakefield DS, Ward M, Miller T, et al. Intensive care unit utilization and interhospital transfers as potential indicators of rural hospital quality. J Rural Health 2004;20:394–400.

75. Rosenberg DI, Moss MM. Guidelines and levels of care for pediatric intensive care units. Crit Care Med 2004;32:2117–27.

76. Merenstein D, Egleston B, Diener-West M. Lengths of stay and costs associated with children's hospitals. Pediatrics 2005;115:839–44.

77. Odetola FO, Gebremariam A, Freed GL. Patient and hospital correlates of clinical outcomes and resource utilization in severe pediatric sepsis. Pediatrics 2007;119:487–94.

78. Gupta RS, Bewtra M, Prosser LA, et al. Predictors of hospital charges for children admitted with asthma. Ambul Pediatr 2006;6:15–20.

79. Dharmar M, Smith AC, Armfield NR, et al. Telemedicine for children in need of intensive care. Pediatr Ann 2009;38:562–6.

80. Reynolds HN, Rogove H, Bander J, et al. A working lexicon for the tele-intensive care unit: we need to define tele-intensive care unit to grow and understand it. Telemed J E Health 2011;17(10):773–83.

81. Marcin JP, Schepps DE, Page KA, et al. The use of telemedicine to provide pediatric critical care consultations to pediatric trauma patients admitted to a remote trauma intensive care unit: a preliminary report. Pediatr Crit Care Med 2004;5:251–6.

82. Marcin JP. Telemedicine in the pediatric intensive care unit. Pediatr Clin North Am 2013;60(3):581–92.

83. Kon AA, Marcin JP. Using telemedicine to improve communication during paediatric resuscitations. J Telemed Telecare 2005;11(5):261–4.

84. Yager PH, Cummings BM, Whalen MJ, et al. Nighttime telecommunication between remote staff intensivists and bedside personnel in a pediatric intensive care unit: a retrospective study. Crit Care Med 2012;40(9):2700–3.
85. Huang T, Moon-Grady A, Traugott C, et al. The availability of telecardiology consultations and transfer patterns from a remote neonatal intensive care unit. J Telemed Telecare 2008;14:244–8.
86. Kon AA, Rich B, Sadorra C, et al. Complex bioethics consultation in rural hospitals: using telemedicine to bring academic bioethicists into outlying communities. J Telemed Telecare 2009;15:264–7.
87. Hall RW, Hall-Barrow J, Garcia-Rill E. Neonatal regionalization through telemedicine using a community-based research and education core facility. Ethn Dis 2010;20(1 Suppl 1). S1-136–S1-140.
88. Kim EW, Teague-Ross T, Greenfield WW, et al. Telemedicine collaboration improves perinatal regionalization and lowers statewide infant mortality. J Perinatol 2013;33(9):725–30.
89. Robie DK, Naulty CM, Parry RL, et al. Early experience using telemedicine for neonatal surgical consultations. J Pediatr Surg 1998;33(7):1172–6 [discussion: 1177].
90. Wenger TL, Gerdes J, Taub K, et al. Telemedicine for genetic and neurologic evaluation in the neonatal intensive care unit. J Perinatol 2014;34(3):234–40.
91. Webb CL, Waugh CL, Grigsby J, et al. Impact of telemedicine on hospital transport, length of stay, and medical outcomes in infants with suspected heart disease: a multicenter study. J Am Soc Echocardiogr 2013;26(9):1090–8.
92. Armfield NR, Donovan T, Bensink ME, et al. The costs and potential savings of telemedicine for acute care neonatal consultation: preliminary findings. J Telemed Telecare 2012;18(8):429–33.
93. Rosenfeld BA, Dorman T, Breslow MJ, et al. Intensive care unit telemedicine: alternate paradigm for providing continuous intensivist care. Crit Care Med 2000;28:3925–31.
94. Breslow MJ, Rosenfeld BA, Doerfler M, et al. Effect of a multiple-site intensive care unit telemedicine program on clinical and economic outcomes: an alternative paradigm for intensivist staffing. Crit Care Med 2004;32:31–8.
95. Thomas EJ, Lucke JF, Wueste L, et al. Association of telemedicine for remote monitoring of intensive care patients with mortality, complications, and length of stay. JAMA 2009;302:2671–8.
96. Franzini L, Sail KR, Thomas EJ, et al. Costs and cost-effectiveness of a telemedicine intensive care unit program in 6 intensive care units in a large health care system. J Crit Care 2011;26:329.e1–6.
97. Nassar BS, Vaughan-Sarrazin MS, Jiang L, et al. Impact of an intensive care unit telemedicine program on patient outcomes in an integrated health care system. JAMA Intern Med 2014;174(7):1160–7.
98. Kohl BA, Fortino-Mullen M, Praestgaard A, et al. The effect of ICU telemedicine on mortality and length of stay. J Telemed Telecare 2012;18:282–6.
99. McCambridge M, Jones K, Paxton H, et al. Association of health information technology and teleintensivist coverage with decreased mortality and ventilator use in critically ill patients. Arch Intern Med 2010;170:648–53.
100. Morrison JL, Cai Q, Davis N, et al. Clinical and economic outcomes of the electronic intensive care unit: results from two community hospitals. Crit Care Med 2010;38:2–8.
101. Lilly CM, Cody S, Zhao H, et al. Hospital mortality, length of stay, and preventable complications among critically ill patients before and after tele-ICU reengineering of critical care processes. JAMA 2011;305:2175–83.

102. Kahn JM. The use and misuse of ICU telemedicine. JAMA 2011;305:2227–8.
103. Lilly CM, McLaughlin JM, Zhao H, et al. A multicenter study of ICU telemedicine reengineering of adult critical care. Chest 2014;145(3):500–7.
104. Young LB, Chan PS, Lu X, et al. Impact of telemedicine intensive care unit coverage on patient outcomes: a systematic review and meta-analysis. Arch Intern Med 2011;171:498–506.
105. Wilcox ME, Adhikari NK. The effect of telemedicine in critically ill patients: systematic review and meta-analysis. Crit Care 2012;16:R127.
106. Smith AC, Armfield NR. A systematic review and meta-analysis of ICU telemedicine reinforces the need for further controlled investigations to assess the impact of telemedicine on patient outcomes. Evid Based Nurs 2011;14(4): 102–3.
107. Kahn JM. Intensive care unit telemedicine: promises and pitfalls. Arch Intern Med 2011;171:495–6.
108. Kumar G, Falk DM, Bonello RS, et al. The costs of critical care telemedicine programs: a systematic review and analysis. Chest 2013;143(1):19–29.
109. Rogove HJ, McArthur D, Demaerschalk BM, et al. Barriers to telemedicine: survey of current users in acute care units. Telemed J E Health 2012;18:48–53.
110. Boots RJ, Singh S, Terblanche M, et al. Remote care by telemedicine in the ICU: many models of care can be effective. Curr Opin Crit Care 2011;17:634–40.
111. Moeckli J, Cram P, Cunningham C, et al. Staff acceptance of a telemedicine intensive care unit program: a qualitative study. J Crit Care 2013;28(6):890–901.
112. Reynolds HN, Bander J, McCarthy M. Different systems and formats for tele-ICU coverage: designing a tele-ICU system to optimize functionality and investment. Crit Care Nurs Q 2012;35:364–77.
113. Rogove H. How to develop a tele-ICU model? Crit Care Nurs Q 2012;35:357–63.
114. Kahn JM, Hill NS, Lilly CM, et al. The research agenda in ICU telemedicine: a statement from the critical care societies collaborative. Chest 2011;140(1): 230–8.

Telemedicine and the Patient with Sepsis

Omar Badawi, PharmD, MPH[a,b,]*, Erkan Hassan, PharmD[a]

KEYWORDS

- Telemedicine • Sepsis • Tele-ICU • Performance improvement • Clinical informatics

KEY POINTS

- Technology can be used to leverage but not replace the need for clinical expertise in the diagnosis, treatment, and assessment of severe sepsis.
- Initial and ongoing proactive screening for severe sepsis is an onerous task that is best managed by leveraging technology for automated screening and remote clinicians to identify potential patients at risk.
- Telemedicine teams can help support bedside personnel improve adherence with sepsis bundles.
- The telemedicine team can use a centralized database to report sepsis performance improvement metrics and trends over time.

INTRODUCTION

Sepsis is a major global public health problem with both a relatively high incidence and mortality rate. The incidence of severe sepsis varies based on the patient population being studied. Severe sepsis may occur in up to 50% to 75% of critically ill patients in many countries, with 50 to 100 cases per 100,000 population.[1,2] Mortality rates for severe sepsis average between 20% and 50%, although these may be declining in recent years.[3,4] The diagnosis of severe sepsis consists of (1) presence of infection, (2) systemic manifestations of inflammation secondary to the infection (sepsis), and (3) organ dysfunction as a result of sepsis.[5]

Although the diagnostic criteria seem rather straightforward, these require human clinical assessment of the patient to make a diagnosis of severe sepsis. At present, a computer does not possess the necessary attributes to meet this goal. Therefore, the best use of automated computer systems at this time seems to be identification of possible patients with severe sepsis as a screening mechanism rather than as a diagnostic function.

Disclosure statement: Dr O. Badawi and Dr E. Hassan are both employees of Philips Healthcare.
[a] Hospital to Home, Philips Healthcare, 217 East Redwood Street, Suite 1900, Baltimore, MD 21202, USA; [b] Department of Pharmacy Practice and Science, University of Maryland School of Pharmacy, Baltimore, MD 21201, USA
* Corresponding author.
E-mail address: omar.badawi@philips.com

Crit Care Clin 31 (2015) 291–304
http://dx.doi.org/10.1016/j.ccc.2014.12.007
0749-0704/15/$ – see front matter © 2015 Elsevier Inc. All rights reserved.

The term telemedicine usually evokes a mental image of computerized monitoring systems, displays, laboratory systems, and radiology information systems, all resulting in medical analog data being converted to digital data. Recently, a variety of approaches and systems for intensive care unit (ICU) telemedicine have evolved.[6] With these technological advances, investigators have reported on the feasibility and outcome of screening and managing the patient in the ICU with severe sepsis via a tele-ICU program.[7,8] Severe sepsis poses numerous interesting factors as a target of improved management and performance via a tele-ICU solution.

There are numerous ways telemedicine can support a therapeutic area, with one of the primary goals being to standardize and promote high reliability for those aspects that are universally accepted. Another (perhaps secondary) goal is to provide a platform for which different approaches can be evaluated. This goal can be reached by creating a standard approach that can be applied reliably, evaluated, and iterated based on findings.

This article focuses on how telemedicine has been applied to the care of the patient with sepsis, the evidence supporting these approaches, and the unchartered applications. These topics are covered through each aspect of septic care by first discussing routine bedside care followed by how telemedicine has been or can be integrated for support. Although management and oversight should be addressed first during the process of implementing a sepsis clinical program, they are discussed here after all aspects of a sepsis program are reviewed, as outlined below.

1. Screening and diagnosis
2. Managing patients with sepsis
    a. Supporting bundle adherence
    b. Therapeutic monitoring
    c. Adverse drug reaction (ADR) monitoring
3. Management and oversight of the entire sepsis program

SCREENING FOR SEPSIS

Screening for sepsis is a critical component to any sepsis program. Active sepsis screening not only improves the timeliness of identifying sepsis but also likely improves the rate at which it is diagnosed.[9] Without a deliberate sepsis screening process, sepsis may not be recognized until patients have progressed to the point of having multiple organ dysfunction. An observational study of 2619 patients in Spanish ICUs found that 78% of cases had 2 or more organ failures present at the time of diagnosis with 58% of the cases already progressing to shock.[10] Similarly, an evaluation of documentation patterns of severe sepsis in a cohort of 664 patients with a severe sepsis diagnosis found that 74% of the cases had cardiovascular dysfunction at the time of diagnosis.[11] Both groups of researchers hypothesized that diagnosis may be delayed in many of these patients yielding high rates of shock, multiple organ failure, and ultimately mortality.

When discussing screening for sepsis, the physical location of the patient within the health system must be the first consideration. Patients can develop sepsis at any point in time, therefore at the time sepsis begins to develop, patients may be

- At home
- Responded to by emergency medical services
- In a primary care clinic
- In a low-acuity health care facility such as a nursing or rehabilitation facility
- In an emergency department (ED)
- In a general hospital ward
- In an ICU

The mechanism of sepsis screening clearly depends on where the patient is physically located, where they are in relation to a transition in care, what data are available, and what technology is available. The most well-known screening criteria for sepsis are the systemic inflammatory response syndrome (SIRS) criteria proposed by Bone and colleagues[12] in 1989. These criteria state that sepsis is the presence of 2 of the 4 SIRS criteria because of an infection, although this has now been amended to included suspected infection. As the presence of an infection is often difficult to assess immediately, the 2 of 4 SIRS criteria has often been used as an initial rule for screening patients for sepsis. The benefit of these criteria is that they are easy to learn, use, replicate, and standardize. Unfortunately, these criteria alone have poor sensitivity and specificity for identifying clinically defined sepsis. Once these criteria are met, 2 determinations still need to be done: (1) is the patient infected and (2) is the presence of SIRS due to the infection? Automating diagnosis is not considered feasible because of the reliance on these clinical definitions; therefore clinicians are required to make the final diagnosis.

More recently, new criteria for sepsis have been proposed, which greatly expand the list of potential SIRS criteria.[5] Patients must have some of the items listed below, which are considered secondary to an infection.[13] Many of these factors are not readily available or known for most patients, and this can lead to underdiagnosis or delays in diagnosis while waiting for results to return (**Box 1**).

All forms of sepsis diagnosis require an infection to be present or suspected to be present. As laboratory data are unlikely to be readily available when dealing with ambulatory or lower-acuity patients, initial screening should focus on determining if the patient has a clinical presentation consistent with infection rather than screening for laboratory markers of systemic inflammation. In ambulatory settings, telemedicine is typically deployed as a consultative model and workflows are minimally different from those of routine care. There are numerous telemedicine models today in which patients can have telephone or video calls with physicians or nurses who can perform the initial screening remotely. Technology can help prompt clinicians to evaluate for SIRS criteria when patients are suspected to have an infection, and assessment of those criteria not requiring invasive tests can be done remotely. Checklists have been used successfully in a variety of clinical settings as a method of improving reliability during periodic events, such as before initiating surgery.[14]

Transitions of care are another example of periodic events that are easily amenable to support tools such as a checklist. Assessing patients remotely during these transitions of care may not change the workflow per se but can provide some distinct advantages of expertise and standardization. For example, every time a patient is admitted to the ED with an infection, a remote consult with an infectious disease or critical care specialist can occur for a formal assessment of sepsis in conjunction with the ED clinician. This process would improve the consistency with which diagnostic criteria are applied. The same argument can be made during all care transitions escalating to a higher level of care such as transitioning from the ED to the general ward or from the general ward to the ICU.

The much more difficult aspect of screening is ongoing screening after a transition in care has occurred. If done manually, this can be time consuming and labor intensive, and although it is very important, it has relatively low yield. An example of this would be if a daily checklist as part of rounds included screening for sepsis. This increased attention would help improve timely diagnosis, but if screening was performed once every 24 hours, it would still lead to potentially large delays in diagnosis and would likely only rarely yield a true new case of sepsis; this is based on the fact that the positive predictive value (PPV) of any screening test is directly related to the

Box 1
Diagnostic criteria for sepsis and severe sepsis

Some of the following must be present secondary to an infection to make the diagnosis of sepsis:

- Fever or hypothermia
- Tachycardia
- Tachypnea
- Altered mental status
- Significant edema or positive fluid balance
- Hyperglycemia in the absence of diabetes
- Leukocytosis or leukopenia
- Elevated levels of plasma C-reactive protein
- Elevated levels of plasma procalcitonin
- Hypotension
- Arterial hypoxemia
- Renal impairment (acute oliguria or rise in levels of serum creatinine)
- Coagulation abnormalities
- Ileus
- Thrombocytopenia
- Hyperbilirubinemia
- Hyperlactatemia
- Decreased capillary refill or mottling

Severe sepsis is defined by sepsis plus at least 1 organ dysfunction secondary to the sepsis:

- Hypotension
- Hyperlactatemia
- Renal injury
- Acute lung injury
- Hyperbilirubinemia
- Thrombocytopenia
- Coagulopathy

Adapted from Levy MM, Fink MP, Marshall JC, et al. 2001 SCCM/ESICM/ACCP/ATS/SIS International Sepsis Definitions Conference. Crit Care Med 2003;31:1252.

prevalence of a disease when sensitivity and specificity are held constant. PPV is the proportion of positive test results that indicate a true positive for disease. For example, if a screening test for sepsis has a sensitivity of 95% and a specificity of 95%, the PPV will be 83% if the disease is relatively common with a prevalence of 20%. However, if the disease is rare and only prevalent in 0.1% of the population being screened, the same test yields a PPV of only 1.9%. Furthermore, the value of a screening tool is obviously only in identifying new cases of sepsis, not cases that the clinical team is currently aware of and actively treating; this is a critical part of the equation because the population being screened for sepsis only involves those not actively being treated for sepsis, and the condition is therefore much rarer than in the entire population being managed.

Case Example

Assume your tele-ICU program is monitoring 100 patients in the ICU and that 15 of these will have an episode of severe sepsis before discharge (ie, cumulative incidence of 15%). If 10 of those cases are admitted for severe sepsis, then there is no value in further screening these patients while they are being treated. Therefore the population of patients that will be screened for severe sepsis in the ICU is only 90, rather than the 100 patients being cared for. Of these 90 patients being screened, only 5 (5.6%) will develop severe sepsis at some point in their ICU stay. Lowering the prevalence even further is the fact that some of those 5 remaining cases of severe sepsis may not have developed yet. Therefore, the prevalence of unrecognized severe sepsis will range somewhere between 0% and 5.6% for the remainder of 90 patients' ICU stay. Even with a remarkably accurate screening tool, the PPV will likely be less than 25% at identifying new cases after admission because of the low prevalence in the cohort of patients being screened. **Fig. 1** illustrates this example for the first 12 sepsis cases identified out of 100 ICU admissions if 10 patients have sepsis on admission and the rest develop sepsis x hours after admission.

Time in the ICU progresses from left to right. The boxes in black reflect the group of patients eligible for future sepsis screening. The patients discussed in gray boxes represent cases of sepsis identified during the current screening process and who will receive treatment. There is no longer any value to screening these patients and therefore they do not contribute to the prevalence calculation for future screening.

Despite these daunting numbers, benefit can be derived from actively screening patients after transitions in care with or without the aid of electronic screening tools. In a report by Rincon and colleagues,[7] remote tele-ICU nurses manually reviewed the medical charts of all patients in the ICU on admission and at least once every 12 hours if they were infected in order to screen for severe sepsis. Cases thought to be new were reviewed with a remote intensivist and then the bedside provider for

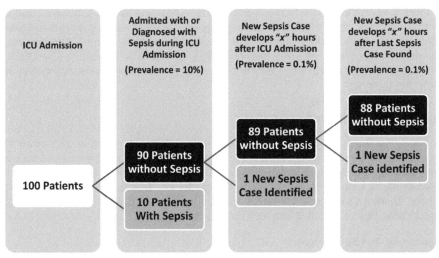

Fig. 1. Example of how the prevalence of new sepsis cases dramatically drops after admission screening.

confirmation. Over the course of 3 years, 211,833 screens were performed on 68,933 patients, which helped identify 5437 cases of severe sepsis. By leveraging the presence of tele-ICU nurses for proactive severe sepsis screening, they were able to significantly improve bundle adherence.[7]

Sepsis is one area in which technology has clearly shown an ability to improve the efficiency with which screening is performed. By automating this process with a tool that has 90% sensitivity and 80% specificity, some tele-ICUs have eliminated the time-intensive process of nurse screening by manually abstracting data with an automated screening tool that continuously evaluates patients to identify those who may have developed sepsis.[15,16]

Automated screening tools have also been managed at the bedside, but the low PPV of sepsis alerts is problematic for bedside providers. Disrupting a physician's time to review an alert that yields sepsis less than 10% of the time is generally considered unacceptable and difficult to integrate into workflow. By leveraging remote clinicians to do the primary evaluation of a highly sensitive screening tool (but with a low PPV), the bedside team can remain focused on routine care while the remote team identifies patients most likely to have sepsis.

Other forms of screening have also been performed in patients not in the ICU. One group of researchers used an internally developed algorithm designed to improve the sensitivity and specificity of the SIRS criteria to identify sepsis in patients not in the ICU.[17] The use of an electronic sepsis alert on patients in the general ward increased therapeutic and diagnostic interventions in patients not critically ill. It should be noted that screening is not sufficient to improve care and some researchers were not able to detect a clinical benefit with introduction of an electronic sepsis screening tool.[18] Great attention must be placed on developing appropriate workflows that maximize the efficiency and optimize the skill set of the team.

Diagnosis must be tightly coupled with screening in any workflow. Telemedicine can play a role in improving diagnosis for sepsis in several scenarios. As discussed earlier, sepsis is a clinical diagnosis and requires human assessment. However, the consistency and reliability of making a sepsis diagnosis may be suboptimal.[10,11] Technology cannot replace this human process, but it can provide a platform to improve the consistency with which the diagnosis is made and reduce delays in diagnosis.[8] Current practice is such that the primary physician determines whether a diagnosis of sepsis should be made, and this leads to the diagnosis being made by physicians with different specialties and varying degrees of expertise and experience. Not only can telemedicine facilitate reducing this variability, but there is a practical benefit to focusing training and education efforts on the fewer remote clinicians rather than all bedside physicians.

MANAGING PATIENTS WITH SEPSIS

In 2002, the Surviving Sepsis Campaign was developed to improve outcomes in sepsis. Large variability in the clinical management of the patient with severe sepsis has resulted in the development of the severe sepsis bundle elements. Originally, there were 6- and 24-hour bundles. In 2013, the guidelines have been revised to 3- and 6-hour bundle elements.[5] Numerous reports have been published demonstrating the positive effects on bundle adherence and mortality.[18–21]

Supporting Bundle Adherence

Telemedicine does not allow for the remote clinician to perform procedures that aid in the completion of the severe sepsis bundle elements (eg, placement of central lines). However, management of severe sepsis, after the diagnosis has been made, is where the clinician can leverage technology to improve outcomes. There are several tasks to be completed within a specified time frame in order to meet the bundle elements. The speed and accuracy of these interventions directly affect the overall outcome of the patient with severe sepsis. In order to accomplish the 3- and 6-hour bundle elements, clinicians must function efficiently and be constantly vigilant of the time constraints. Although not frequently addressed in the literature, determination and establishment of time zero (T-zero) is critical because all future elements are relative to this time. The definition of T-zero changes based on the location of diagnosis.[13] The clinician needs to be aware of 2 possible T-zero determinations based on patient location at the time of diagnosis. Most patients with severe sepsis are admitted from the ED; in these patients, T-zero is defined as the time of emergency room triage as opposed to the onset of clinical manifestations consistent with severe sepsis. The remaining patients with severe sepsis are identified while in the hospital, either in the ICU or in the non-ICU environment (ie, patients in the general ward). Severe sepsis T-zero in the hospitalized patient is the time when clinical manifestations meeting the definition of severe sepsis first occur, which may be different from the time of identification by a clinician.[13] Although telemedicine may be used to screen patients for severe sepsis, clinical evaluation remains the optimal method for assessing and determining the appropriate T-zero. However, once established, the technology associated with telemedicine can help drive the bundles in many ways. The 3- and 6-hour bundle times of completion can be easily calculated and displayed for the telehealth center clinicians to monitor while the bedside team hurriedly moves through the chaos of a typical ICU day. Improved timeliness of interventions can be tracked by a timer alerting the clinician when the 3- and 6-hour bundle times are closing and the remaining items to be achieved within the bundle. Although a 6-hour protocol of early goal-directed therapy (EGDT) has recently been called into question, early recognition and treatment of the patient with severe sepsis remains the ideal approach.[22,23] To achieve EGDT typically, at least 2 L of crystalloid needs to be administered over the 6-hour period. Monitoring the initial resuscitation volume infusion and the subsequent hemodynamic results (or lack thereof) could be a function of the remote telehealth clinician. Since the publication of the original Surviving Sepsis Campaign in 2004, a protocoled approach to the management of the patient with severe sepsis has been advocated and shown to improve outcomes. Recently, the ProCESS (Protocolized Care for Early Septic Shock) trial has questioned the value of EGDT in the management of the patient with severe sepsis.[22] Regardless of the final role of EGDT, the other protocol processes (ie, early recognition of and antibiotic treatment of sepsis) are still deemed of value in the management of the patient with severe sepsis. Current recommendations are for antimicrobials to be administered within the first hour of recognition of severe sepsis.[5] The 1 hour time to antimicrobial administration was from data of 17,990 patients demonstrating a statistically significant increase in the probability of death associated with a delay in antibiotic administration after the first hour. In addition, each hour delay resulted in a linear increase in the risk of mortality.[24] The 1-hour time window is not consistently the current standard of clinical practice. Median time from ED triage to antibiotic administration in patients with severe sepsis or septic shock has been documented to be close to 2 hours with only 27% of patients receiving antibiotics within 1 hour.[25,26] Although antibiotic timing is important, a second consideration is the appropriateness of the antibiotic regimen. Failure to cover the appropriate organism or organisms would be equivalent to delayed antibiotic administration. The causative organisms for sepsis have evolved over the past 2 decades. The causative organism of sepsis may be bacteria (gram-positive organisms now exceeding gram-negative organisms), fungus, as well as virus. Fungal infections are growing at a larger rate than bacterial causes.[27] The prominent annual cause of sepsis in the United States in 2000 was gram-positive bacteria in 52.1% of cases, followed by gram-negative bacteria at 37.6%. Fungal infections caused sepsis in 4.6% of the cases. However, over a 22-year period, the number of cases caused by fungal organisms increased by 207%, exceeding the general increase in incidence of either gram-positive or gram-negative organisms.[3] Although, gram-negative bacteremia is associated with a higher mortality than gram-positive bacteremia, approximately one-third of patients with severe sepsis never have positive result of blood cultures.[28] The importance of rapid, accurate antimicrobial treatment is counterbalanced by the increased incidence of bacterial resistance over time. Increasing hospital-acquired infections coupled with broad-spectrum antibiotic use in the critically ill patients who remain in the ICU for longer periods has most likely contributed to the increased resistance rates.[29,30] Applying technology to the antibiotic portion of the severe sepsis bundles would involve at least 3 major components. These components are (1) patient-specific microbiology results, (2) local antibiotic guidelines/policies, and (3) unit-specific antibiotic susceptibility data for common pathogens. These data may not be easily accessible. Specific microbiology results must provide just-in-time results. Factoring in 2 sets of blood cultures, cultures from other bodily sites, and the frequent laboratory reports of pending reports, it would not be difficult to envision several nuisance alerts because the results for every sample are reported. In addition, this requirement would not be of value in the one-third of patients without positive results of cultures. Technological approaches such as an antibiotic-prescribing computer-based decision support (CDS) system can address the major areas outlined above. One such system as described by Sintchenko and colleagues[31] demonstrates that microbiology results are the most commonly accessed data at 53% of the time the system was used. Antibiotics guidelines were the second most commonly accessed data, but far removed at only 22.5% of the time. The use of the antibiotic-prescribing CDS resulted in a reduction in antibiotic use in the ICU with changes in patterns of antibiotic use. Total consumption of β-lactamase-resistant penicillins and vancomycin had the most significant reduction in use ($P<.05$). In addition, telemedicine approaches could help clinicians ensure appropriate antibiotic administration in a timely manner relative to T-zero, as well as identify cases when the antibiotics were delayed. Once final culture results are available, the tele-ICU can aid in the antibiotic streamlining process in a timely manner.

Therapeutic Monitoring

In addition to supporting bundle adherence, monitoring of patients with severe sepsis involves 2 major areas: therapeutic monitoring to determine if the patient is responding to current therapy and toxicity monitoring to ensure that current therapies are not resulting in adverse events. Although current advances allow for technology to aid in these efforts, clinical assessments by experts remain essential.

Patients with severe sepsis with persistent or refractory hypotension or tissue hypoperfusion despite adequate fluid resuscitation meet the definition of septic shock. Therapy at this time should progress to vasopressor therapy; the role of telemedicine then shifts from timing of initiation of therapy to hemodynamic therapeutic monitoring. This monitoring is done to ensure single (eg, norepinephrine, grade 1B) or when appropriate, double vasopressors (eg, norepinephrine with epinephrine, grade 2B, or vasopressin, ungraded) achieve a mean arterial pressure (MAP) of at least 65 mm Hg. In addition, with ongoing signs of hypoperfusion despite achieving adequate intravascular volume and an adequate MAP greater than or equal to 65 mm Hg, improved oxygen tissue delivery would be warranted. The 2012 revised Surviving Sepsis Campaign bundles call for MAP of at least 65 mm Hg, central venous pressure (CVP) of at least 8 mm Hg, and central venous oxygen saturation ($Scvo_2$) of at least 70%.[5] The serum lactate concentration may also need to be remeasured if the initial value was elevated. The tele-ICU clinician can help monitor therapeutic responsiveness and notify the bedside team to alter the patients' care plan to aid achieving adherence with the 6-hour severe sepsis bundles.

Most studies indicate that even with maximal therapy, mortality from severe sepsis remains high.[19–21] This persistent high mortality rate despite adequate therapy indicates that current modalities will most likely not reduce mortality from severe sepsis to 0. Therefore, ongoing therapeutic monitoring to determine which patients are responding, and potentially even more important, which patients are not responding to therapy is an important consideration. Monitoring for therapeutic benefit involves assessing the clinical course of the patient to ensure progressive improvement. Initial monitoring may involve objective physiologic data, and this includes, but is not limited to, appropriate antibiotic selections based on likely and documented microbiological results, improved trends in temperature, white blood cell counts, serum lactate clearance, as well as reversal with improvements in respiratory and/or hemodynamic findings. Recently, several biomarkers have been highlighted as a tool not only in the early diagnosis but also as a possible mechanism to monitor the progression of the disease. The effectiveness of these biomarkers is typically limited because of the heterogeneity in the amount of physiologic inflammatory and immune response processes in patients with severe sepsis.[32] Technology associated with telemedicine including laboratory, vital sign, and microbiological interfaces may provide these data to the clinician to assess in relation to therapy. However, this should not be the sole determining factor. As indicated earlier, up to one-third of microbiological results may be negative. Although serum lactate clearance data may prove beneficial in determining early response rates, other physiologic variables may have delayed responses. For these reasons, clinical assessment of the patient plays a vital role in determining if the patient is having a favorable clinical response.

Adverse Drug Reaction Monitoring

As with the treatment of any disease state, patients being treated for severe sepsis should be monitored to quickly detect the development of any adverse drug reactions (ADRs) based on their therapeutic regimen. ADRs account for 4.2% to 30% of hospitalizations per year in the United States and are associated with increased length of stay and costs.[33] The incidence of fatal ADRs in hospitalized patients has been estimated at 0.32%.[34] Antimicrobials have been reported to be the second highest cause of ADR-related costs.[35] ADR severity is assessed in a subjective manner based on treatment approach and outcome. The definition used to assess ADR severity ranges from mild to fatal and is outlined in **Table 1**.[34]

It is difficult to diagnose a drug hypersensitivity reaction. The facts that various drugs can elicit a wide variety of immune-mediated reactions, assessment can be subjective, and there is always a lack of need to discontinue therapy make it extremely difficult to program electronic alerts for the identification of ADRs via a telemedicine solution. A telemedicine solution could be used to address areas that may prevent an ADR.[34] Even with such technological assistance, the clinician should not solely assume that a positive finding is a definitive ADR, but rather rely on clinical assessment for conclusion (**Box 2**).

Table 1
ADR severity

Severity	Definition
Mild	Uncomplicated; not requiring treatment with drug discontinuation not necessary; does not prolong hospital stay
Moderate	Requires treatment or prolongs hospitalization by at least 1 d; drug discontinuation not necessary; some but not all of the mild criteria and none of the severe criteria
Severe	Potentially life threatening; drug discontinuation required; treatment of ADR is permanently disabling, requires intensive medical care, or takes longer than 14 d to recover
Fatal	ADR directly or indirectly contributes to a patient's death

Adapted from Pourpak Z, Mohammad R, Fazlollahi R, et al. Understanding adverse drug reactions and drug allergies: principles, diagnosis and treatment aspects. Recent Pat Inflamm Allergy Drug Discov 2008;2:33; with permission.

MANAGEMENT AND OVERSIGHT OF THE ENTIRE SEPSIS PROGRAM

Guidelines or protocols alone have little impact on bedside behavior to improve clinical outcomes. In order for a hospital-based performance improvement initiative to improve outcomes, a formal program consisting of a multiprofessional team with defined roles and responsibilities, formal educational sessions, preaudit and postaudit data, and feedback to all parties is necessary.[36,37] The team should minimally include physicians, nurses, pharmacists, respiratory, laboratory, and clinical educators as well as representatives from the ICU, general ward, and EDs. Representation should not only be at the manager or director level but also should include those clinicians actually performing the tasks from both day and evening shifts. Once the roles and responsibilities of all parties are defined, the metrics to be collected, which determine the success of the program, should be clearly identified and agreed upon by all stakeholders.

Once each team member's roles and responsibilities have been defined, educational sessions can be designed and implemented. The objectives of the educational sessions are to review screening methodologies, team members' roles, specific treatment protocols developed, and any other site-specific considerations. Although live educational sessions are preferred, these may be supplemented by telelearning methodologies to ensure that all clinicians are trained and/or available to review after a training session as needed.

Box 2
Areas telemedicine could address in an attempt to minimize ADRs

- Drug use appropriate for patient diagnosis
- Dose, route, and frequency of administration appropriate for patients' weight, age, and diagnosis
- Ordering of laboratory test results and other monitoring for each drug
- Presence of allergic reaction (or previous reaction) to drug (or class)
- Drug-drug or drug-food interaction warnings

Adapted from Pourpak Z, Mohammad R, Fazlollahi R, et al. Understanding adverse drug reactions and drug allergies: principles, diagnosis and treatment aspects. Recent Pat Inflamm Allergy Drug Discov 2008;2:24–46; with permission.

Data collection should occur on a continuous basis, not just Monday through Friday. Once the program is implemented, a review to ensure that the data are being collected as originally designed should be made relatively quickly (ie, 2–4 weeks after initiation). The primary purpose of this review is to determine what is working and what is not working and provide a mechanism to iterate the process. For the activities that are not fully functioning, the primary question should be to determine if the original work-flows were created incorrectly or if further educational sessions are required for everyone to fully understand their roles and responsibilities. Adjustments can then be made and reevaluated. The need for adjustments should not be considered failures of the design, but rather as an expected part of the process of implementing and managing a program.

Improved compliance with the severe sepsis bundle elements has been shown to decrease mortality in this patient population.[18–21] Therefore, to improve patient outcomes as well as assess efficacy of a sepsis management program, compliance with accepted severe sepsis bundles should be considered a mandatory monitoring function. The time limits associated with bundle compliance make achieving the individual components and entire bundle a difficult task. Telemedicine alone cannot achieve complete bundle compliance determination; rather a combined effort of clinical input and assessment along with technology provides the most efficient approach.

As previously stated, one of the most important metrics in the evaluation of the patient with severe sepsis is the determination of the onset of the sepsis syndrome. Although technology is extremely efficient at reviewing a large amount of data, pinpointing the time of the development of severe sepsis (and hence the diagnosis of severe sepsis) is purely a clinical determination beyond the reach of commonly available technology today. Therefore, the onset of severe sepsis (defined as T-zero), which begins the time frame for bundle completion, can only be accomplished with clinical input. Once established, it is not too difficult to envision an electronic system that can help the clinician monitor the necessary steps to initiate and the attainable end points in the patient with severe sepsis in order to achieve all bundle elements in a timely manner. Examples of these functions, many of which can be efficiently managed via telemedicine, are provided below.

Functions Technology Can Help Monitor in the Patient with Severe Sepsis

1. Fluid resuscitation volume based on patient body weight should be calculated, and it should be monitored whether the calculated volume is infused within the appropriate time frame.
2. Once T-zero is identified, the system should track the time and progress to ensure that necessary bundle elements are achieved.
3. Care limitations designated for the patient should be identified and notified to the clinician.
4. Laboratory interfaces should autopopulate the following available fields:
    a. Lactate: initial and subsequent values with clearance calculations
    b. Blood culture results (including fungal assays): within-bundle time limits
    c. Antibiotics: specific agents and within-bundle time limits
    d. Procalcitonin concentrations
5. Cardiorespiratory parameters
    a. MAP
    b. CVP
    c. Vasoactive support
    d. Svo_2 or $Scvo_2$

6. Time to attain 3- and 6-hour bundle elements
   a. Were all elements attained within the specified time frame
   b. If not, specify which elements were not met

Educational efforts must be ongoing to reinforce early identification and treatment protocols of the patient with severe sepsis. These efforts can be attained via electronic learning modules as enduring learning materials. In addition, as clinical staff turnover or new staff are hired, ongoing educational sessions will be required to maintain high performance.

With the institution of telemedicine technology as indicated above, periodic performance metrics can be reviewed as desired through the electronic database query. The use of technology allows performance to be plotted and displayed over any time period with a tabular or graphic display. In addition, detailed analysis can be reviewed based on the ICU or the provider to identify high performers and highlight areas needing improvement. Finally, the displays can aid in identifying the reasons for not meeting the 3- and 6-hour bundles with attention to address these deficiencies and improve outcomes. Improvement of clinical programs requires ongoing and consistent data collection, measurement of metrics, and feedback to the team for continual improvement. By integrating telemedicine to the process, the telemedicine team becomes ideally situated to manage these processes efficiently and support the needs of the bedside team.

SUMMARY

Sepsis and severe sepsis are relatively common in the ICU and are associated with high mortality. Telemedicine can support nearly all facets of sepsis management to improve the quality and reliability of care as well as serve as a platform for sepsis program management. Proactive, continuous screening is difficult to implement without telemedicine support because of the low prevalence of unrecognized severe sepsis and the subsequent low PPV of virtually all screening criteria. Once screening is performed, telemedicine can allow remote specialists to support diagnosis and management in a variety of workflows. Screening for severe sepsis during transitions of care can be accomplished with and without telemedicine support, but improved standardization of how sepsis diagnostic criteria are applied can be achieved through telemedicine support. Remote clinicians can also support the bedside staff by helping improve adherence with bundle elements and monitoring for therapeutic response and ADRs. Having a comprehensive approach for implementation and management of a sepsis program is critical to ensure continuous performance improvement, and a telemedicine team is well-suited to support program oversight.

REFERENCES

1. Vincent JL, Rello J, Marshall J, et al. International study of the prevalence and outcomes of infection in intensive care units. JAMA 2009;302:2323–9.
2. Danai P, Martin GS. Epidemiology of sepsis: recent advances. Curr Infect Dis Rep 2005;7:329–34.
3. Martin GS. Sepsis, severe sepsis and septic shock: changes in incidence, pathogens and outcomes. Expert Rev Anti Infect Ther 2012;10:701–6.
4. Kaukonen K, Bailey M, Suzuki S, et al. Mortality related to severe sepsis and septic shock among critically ill patients in Australia and New Zealand, 2000-2012. JAMA 2014;311(13):1308–16. http://dx.doi.org/10.1001/jama.2014.2637.

5. Delinger RP, Levy MM, Rhodes A, et al. Surviving sepsis campaign: international guidelines for management of severe sepsis and septic shock: 2012. Crit Care Med 2013;41:580–637.
6. Reynolds HN, Rogove H, Bander J, et al. A working lexicon for the tele-Intensive Care Unit: we need to define tele-Intensive Care Unit to grow and understand it. Telemed J E Health 2011;17:773–83.
7. Rincon TA, Bourke G, Seiver A. Standardizing sepsis screening and management via a tele-ICU program improves patient care. Telemed J E Health 2011;17(7): 560–4.
8. Croft CA, Moore FA, Efron PA, et al. Computer versus paper system for recognition and management of sepsis in surgical intensive care. J Trauma Acute Care Surg 2014;76:311–9.
9. Steinman M, Abreu Filho CA, Andrade A, et al. Implementation of a sepsis protocol in a community hospital using a Telemedicine Program. Crit Care 2013; 17(Suppl 2):P272.
10. Blanco J, Muriel-Bombín A, Sagredo V, et al. Incidence, organ dysfunction and mortality in severe sepsis: a Spanish multicentre study. Crit Care 2008;12(6): R158.
11. Badawi O, Bress A, Zubrow M, et al. Severe sepsis (SS) is underreported in the ICU. 2008 SCCM annual congress poster presentation. Crit Care Med 2007; 35(12 Suppl):A256.
12. Bone RC, Fischer CJ Jr, Clemmer TP, et al. Sepsis syndrome: a valid clinical entity. Crit Care Med 1989;17:389–93.
13. Levy MM, Fink MP, Marshall JC, et al. 2001 SCCM/ESICM/ACCP/ATS/SIS International Sepsis Definitions Conference. Crit Care Med 2003;31:1250–6.
14. Gawande A. The checklist manifesto: how to get things right. New York: Henry Holt & Company; 2010.
15. Jenkins CL, Hassan E, Maxwell DK, et al. Improved screening and management of severe sepsis (SS): combining an integrated multidisciplinary team and technology. Crit Care Med 2009;37(12 Suppl):A738.
16. Badawi O, Fromm R, Rincon T, et al. Using annotated electronic patient data to develop a predictive model for identifying severe sepsis. Crit Care Med 2009; 37(12 Suppl):A224.
17. Sawyer AM, Deal EN, Labelle AJ, et al. Implementation of a real-time computerized sepsis alert in nonintensive care unit patients. Crit Care Med 2011;39(3): 469–73.
18. Hooper MH, Weavind L, Wheeler AP, et al. Randomized trial of automated, electronic monitoring to facilitate early detection of sepsis in the intensive care unit. Crit Care Med 2012;40(7):2096–101.
19. Barochia AV, Cui X, Vitberg D, et al. Bundled care for septic shock: an analysis of clinical trials. Crit Care Med 2010;38:668–78.
20. Castellanos-Ortega A, Suberviola B, Garcia-Astudillo LA, et al. Impact of the surviving sepsis campaign protocols on hospital length of stay and mortality in septic shock patients. Results of a three year follow-up quasi-experimental study. Crit Care Med 2010;38:1036–43.
21. Van Zanten AR, Brinkman S, Arbous S, et al. Guideline bundle adherence and mortality in severe sepsis and septic shock. Crit Care Med 2014;42(8):1890–8.
22. The ProCESS Investigators. A randomized trial of protocol-based care for early septic shock. N Engl J Med 2014;370(18):1683–93.
23. Lilly CM. The ProCESS trial – a new era of sepsis management. N Engl J Med 2014;370(18):1750–1.

24. Ferrer R, Martin-Loeches I, Phillips G, et al. Empiric antibiotic treatment reduces mortality in severe sepsis and septic shock from the first hour: results from a guideline-based performance improvement program. Crit Care Med 2014; 42(8):1749–55.
25. Puskarich MA, Trzeciak S, Shapiro N, et al. Association between timing of antibiotic administration and mortality from septic shock in patients treated with a quantitative resuscitation protocol. Crit Care Med 2011;39:2066–71.
26. Gaieski DF, Mikkelsen ME, Band RA, et al. Impact of time to antibiotics on survival in patients with severe sepsis or septic shock in whom early goal directed therapy was initiated in the emergency department. Crit Care Med 2010;38:1045–53.
27. Martin GS, Mannino DM, Eaton S, et al. The epidemiology of sepsis in the United States from 1979 through 2000. N Engl J Med 2003;348(16):1546–54.
28. Mayr FB, Yende S, Angus DC. Epidemiology of severe sepsis. Virulence 2014;5: 4–11.
29. Reacher MH, Shah A, Livermore DM, et al. Bacteremia and antibiotic resistance of its pathogens reported in England and Wales between 1990 and 1998; trend analysis. BMJ 2000;320:213–6.
30. Carler J, Ben AA, Chalfine A. Epidemiology ad control of antibiotic resistance in the intensive care unit. Curr Opin Infect Dis 2004;17:309–16.
31. Sintchenko V, Iredell JR, Gilbert GL, et al. Handheld computer based decision support reduces patient length of stay and antibiotic prescribing in critical care. J Am Med Inform Assoc 2005;12:398–402.
32. Samrai RS, Zingarelli B, Wong HR. Role of biomarkers in sepsis care. Shock 2013;40:358–65.
33. Sultana J, Cutroneo P, Trifiro G. Clinical and economic burden of adverse drug reactions. J Pharmacol Pharmacother 2013;4(suppl 1):S73–7.
34. Pourpak Z, Mohammad R, Fazlollahi R, et al. Understanding adverse drug reactions and drug allergies: principles, diagnosis and treatment aspects. Recent Pat Inflamm Allergy Drug Discov 2008;2:24–46.
35. White TJ, Arakelian A, Rho JP. Counting the costs of drug-related adverse events. Pharmacoeconomics 1999;15:445–58.
36. Schorr CA, Zanotti S, Dellinger RP. Severe sepsis and septic shock. Management and performance improvement. Virulence 2014;5:190–9.
37. Schorr CA, Dellinger RP. Performance improvement in the management of sepsis. Crit Care Clin 2009;25:857–67.

The Impact of Telemedicine in Cardiac Critical Care

Jayashree Raikhelkar, MD[a,*], Jayant K. Raikhelkar, MD[b]

KEYWORDS

- Telemedicine • Cardiac care • Heart failure • Telecardiology • Echocardiogram
- Electrocardiogram

KEY POINTS

- Telecardiology is one of the fastest growing fields in telemedicine.
- Tele-coronary care unit (tele-CCU) connects the remote cardiologist to the cardiac care unit for consultation.
- Tele-electrocardiogram (tele-ECG) allows for prehospital triage and thrombolysis in patients with ST segment elevation myocardial infarction (STEMI).
- Tele-echocardiogram (tele-echo) and tele-heart failure monitoring include teleconsultation for congenital heart disease and the remote monitoring of heart failure patients.

Telemedicine was recognized in the 1970s as a legitimate entity for applying the use of modern information and communications technologies to the delivery of health services.[1] The earliest mention of telemedicine in cardiology can be traced back to early twentieth century when electrocardiographic data were first transmitted over telephonic wires.[2] Telecardiology is one of the fastest growing fields in telemedicine. The advancement of technologies and Web-based applications has allowed better transmission of health care delivery. Although improvements in cardiac care have led to a substantial decline in cardiac mortality over the last 50 years, cardiovascular diseases are still the leading cause of death in the United States. It is estimated that more than 2000 Americans die of cardiovascular disease every day.[3] Increases in life expectancy have led to concomitant increases in the prevalence of coronary artery disease and chronic heart failure. It is hoped that the rapid developments in telecardiology will benefit this increasing population of patients and play an important role in further improvements cardiovascular

Disclosure: The authors have nothing to disclose.
[a] Department of Anesthesiology and Critical Care, Emory University School of Medicine, 1364 Clifton Road Northeast, Atlanta, GA 30322, USA; [b] Department of Cardiovascular Medicine, University Hospitals Case Medical Center, Case Western Reserve University, 11100 Euclid Avenue, Cleveland, OH 44106, USA
* Corresponding author.
E-mail address: jraikhelkar@yahoo.com

Crit Care Clin 31 (2015) 305–317
http://dx.doi.org/10.1016/j.ccc.2014.12.008
0749-0704/15/$ – see front matter © 2015 Elsevier Inc. All rights reserved.

outcomes into the twenty-first century.[4] This article discusses current advancements, and the scope of telemedicine in cardiology and its application to the critically ill.

Current telemedicine applications include:

- Tele–coronary care unit (tele-CCU): telecardiologist and teleconsultation in the cardiac care unit
- Tele-electrocardiogram (tele-ECG): prehospital electrocardiogram (ECG) triage and thrombolysis in patients with ST segment elevation myocardial infarction (STEMI)
- Tele-echocardiogram: teleconsultation for congenital heart disease and valvular disease
- Tele–heart failure monitoring, including telephonic and physiologic monitoring

TELE–CORONARY CARE UNIT

Several clinical trials have studied the tele–intensive care unit (tele-ICU) model. Various studies have determined that, if implemented properly, tele-ICU can reduce mortality, length of stay, and complication rates, and improve best-practice adherence.[5,6] Tele-ICU technology allows continuous secure transmission of patients' vital signs from an intensive care unit (ICU) to a monitoring center in real time. In addition, monitoring center staff provide teleconsultation and support to bedside physicians and nurses by continuous surveillance and 24-hour alert system. Tele-ICU consultation in the CCU allows continuous monitoring of vital signs, ECG, blood pressure waveforms, oxygen saturation, pulmonary artery catheter waveforms, as well as respiration and body temperature. This process also allows real-time communication and teleconsultation with cardiologists. The feasibility of this concept was studied by Nikus and colleagues.[7] In the Finnish study, remote surveillance of the CCU and cardiology ward was performed by a telecardiologist who had access to electronic medical records. The telecardiologist role was supportive, and this person was available for consultation and emergencies. The remote access of hospital intranet and server applications proved reliable and technically feasible. The study indicated a potential for reducing the delay for diagnostic and therapeutic interventions.[7]

Early diagnosis of acute myocardial infarction and appropriate reperfusion by means of percutaneous coronary angioplasty (percutaneous coronary intervention [PCI]) or thrombolysis has been shown to reduce morbidity and mortality, especially in the setting of STEMI.[8,9] The 2013 American Heart Association/American College of Cardiology STEMI guidelines reinforced the need for regional medical systems to provide reperfusion therapy as rapidly as possible.[10] Much attention is being paid to the concept of prehospital thrombolysis en route to the CCU (**Fig. 1**).[11,12]

Teleconsultation and remote interaction of a paramedic with a cardiologist available in a CCU holds great promise to reduce delay and increase patient survival.[13] Teleconsultation with the support of wireless and mobile technology additionally allows monitoring and surveillance during transport.[14] Smartphone technology also allows highly accurate interpretation of angiographic lesions[15] and may also serve as a supplementary tool for emergency situations in the critically ill.

Telecardiology currently encompasses a wide variety of applications, including the monitoring of cardiac rhythm and function remotely with software technology. Two of the most important tools within the cardiologist domain are the 12-lead ECG and the two-dimensional and three-dimensional echocardiogram. With wireless technology, cardiologists can remotely access information from patient records and offer timely diagnostic and treatment recommendations.

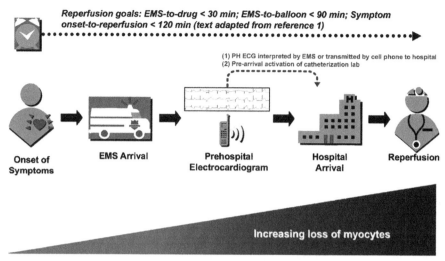

Fig. 1. Reperfusion time goals for patients with STEMI. EMS, emergency medical service; PH, prehospital. (*From* Ting HH, Krumholz HM, Bradley EH, et al. Implementation and integration of prehospital ECGs into systems of care for acute coronary syndrome: a scientific statement from the American Heart Association Interdisciplinary Council on Quality of Care and Outcomes Research, Emergency Cardiovascular Care Committee, Council on Cardiovascular Nursing, and Council on Clinical Cardiology. Circulation 2008;118:1066–79; with permission. © 2008 American Heart Association, Inc.)

ELECTROCARDIOGRAM TELEMONITORING

One of the most important applications of telecardiology is the ability to transmit a recorded ECG to a cardiologist for evaluation. In 3G (third-generation) wireless technology, ECG transmission can occur with the use of mobile phones/tablets at home. The data are delivered via Bluetooth to the hospital.[16] ECG transmission can occur without Internet access as well. Technology has been developed to record ECG signals as audio inputs. This input is transmitted to a hospital with a landline or mobile phone. This technology has allowed patients without Internet access, such as those in rural areas, the ability to record and transmit data to specialized centers. One of the deficiencies of this method is the weak signal quality that may be generated.[17,18] With the advent of 3G technology and transmission control protocol/internet protocol (TCP/IP), ECG transmission has become reliable and the signal quality is enhanced.[19]

Clinical trials related to tele-ECG monitoring have proved its applicability in a real-world setting. Because the time to reperfusion is crucial to improving prognosis in patients with acute myocardial infarction, there have been many studies of prehospital ECG interpretation and early triage of patients with myocardial infarction before reaching the hospital.

Brunetti and colleagues[20] reported preliminary data with respect to prehospital ECG triage in patients with STEMI. In this single-center study, patients with STEMI transferred by regional emergency medical service (EMS) were enrolled in the study. Patient were randomized to receive prehospital ECG triage by telecardiology support and directly transferred to cardiac catheterization for primary PCI or transferred to the emergency department where the diagnosis would be made. Times to balloon and PCI treatment (85% vs 35%; *P*<.001; +141%) were significantly shorter in patients triaged with telecardiology ECG in the EMS registry, in both short-distance and long-distance groups versus controls.[20] In the MonAMI (MonashHEART Acute Myocardial Infarction) study,[21] prehospital ECG triage and activation of the emergency room infarct team resulted in more patients achieving guideline recommendations. Rasmussen and colleagues[22] showed that almost 90% of patients living within 95 km, with prehospital diagnosis and triage of STEMI, could be treated with primary PCI within 120 minutes.

MORTALITIES AND LEFT VENTRICLE FUNCTION

Mortalities have been studied with respect to prehospital triage. Sivagangabalan and colleagues[23] found that ambulance field triage versus emergency room triage for patients with STEMI significantly reduced door-to-balloon times (P<.001) and 30-day mortality, and preserved left ventricular ejection fraction. Field triage decreased revascularization times, and improved early survival. Other investigators have shown that ambulance transmission of electrocardiographic data and triage benefits long-term (1 year) survival as well. Chan and colleagues[24] found that prehospital triage was an independent predictor for survival at 1 year (hazard ratio [HR], 0.37; 95% confidence interval [CI], 0.18–0.75; P = .006).

Concerns have arisen in the cardiology community regarding the accuracy of clinical diagnosis of STEMI with minimal clinical information during telemedicine consultation. A great emphasis is placed on the rapid diagnosis and triage of patients with ECG interpretation when there is scanty history. McCabe and colleagues'[25] study of physician accuracy emphasizes this fact. In this cross-sectional study, there is significant physician disagreement in interpreting ECGs that are concerning for STEMI, and poor agreement for ECG interpretation among specialties. Even after adjusting for experience, there was no significant difference in the odds of accurate interpretation alone, thus indicating that ECGs should not be the only diagnostic test.

Cost-effective of ECG telemedicine is not well studied. Some of the first data on the issue are from an observational study by Brunetti and colleagues.[26] The cost analysis is an observational study based in the Apulia region in Italy. Patients who called the local EMS during 2012 and underwent prehospital triage with telemedicine ECG in cases of suspected acute cardiac disease were included. The ECGs were read remotely by a cardiologist. The cost of usual care versus this method of triage was calculated. Although the cost was calculated and value added tax was not considered, there was a potential saving in presumed lives per year saved and cost per quality-adjusted life year gained.[26]

ECHOTELEMEDICINE

Echocardiography is a vital tool for cardiologists to evaluate ventricular function and valvular disease in the critically ill. Progressive telemedicine technology has a great potential to improve access to specialists in the ICU.

The first mention of interpretation of echocardiography by telemedicine support was in the 1980s, by Finley and colleagues.[27] In 1987 they established a real-time pediatric echocardiography service at a tertiary care center with service to regional hospitals. The system of transmission used was dial-up broadband video transmission. About 70% of the studies were urgent examinations. A comparison between transmitted images and bedside in-person images showed few differences in diagnoses and unnecessary transfers. In 1996, Trippi and colleagues[28] described the use of tele-echocardiography in emergency consultation telemedicine. In their prospective study, urgent echocardiograms were performed off hours (nights, weekends, holidays) assessing for ventricular function, ischemia, valvular disease and so forth. Interpretations of the echocardiograms were compared with interpretations made by reviewing videotapes in a blinded manner. Off-site echocardiographers reviewed the images in a cine-loop format transferred to home laptop computers. Abnormalities were identified in more than 80% of the studies, including wall motion abnormalities, pulmonary hypertension, aortic dissection, valvular dysfunction, and tamponade. Telemedicine and videotape interpretations correlated 99% of the time and the time to generate official echocardiogram reports were reduced significantly. In the same year, Trippi and colleagues[29,30] also performed dobutamine stress echocardiography on 26 patients in emergency rooms admitted for chest pain who were considered low risk for myocardial infarction. The studies (echocardiography cine-loops and ECG tracings) were interpreted by an off-site cardiologist. The images were transmitted to the laptop computer of the cardiologist by traditional phone line linked to a computer modem. Myocardial infarction was ruled out in 25 of the 26 patients.

Recent advances in wireless and smartphone technology have led to echocardiographic interpretation with mobile-to-mobile consultation with predictable accuracy.[31,32]

Pediatric cardiology has been the first field to embrace the concept of tele-echocardiography. Many neonates in small towns and rural areas do not have access to pediatric sonographers or cardiologists. This lack of access may cause a considerable delay in diagnosis. Perhaps the severe shortage of specialists in the field has preempted the early development of telemedicine services. Accurate remote diagnosis and the exclusion of congenital heart disease in patients has had an impact on treatment plans and may produce cost savings by reducing transport needs and unnecessary work-up.[33–35]

One obvious limitation of tele-echocardiography is that a skilled operator is required for proper ultrasonography image acquisition, and the quality of the examination depends heavily on the operator's skills. To overcome this issue, Courreges and colleagues[36] developed and studied a robotic teleultrasonography system (OTELO). It consists of 2 stations, an expect station where the sonographer controls a virtual probe, and a patient station consisting of a real probe held by a lightweight robot. The real probe is positioned on the patient. A total of 52 patients had ultrasonography examinations at 2 different hospitals. The diagnosis obtained with the remote scanning system agreed in at least 80% of the cases with the diagnosis made by conventional scanning. Disagreements with the final diagnosis occurred with lesions caused by low resolutions, suboptimal scanning, and inadequate image acquisition.

Recent technology allows live streaming of echocardiographic imaging and simultaneous video conferencing over the Web. The EchoCart by StatVideo[37] permits video communication between caregivers/families with physicians who can guide the imaging procedure, facilitating understanding about the patient. Because the streaming is over the Web, there is a cost saving as well.

In spite of limitations, real-time tele-echocardiography has been effective in assisting with challenging cases requiring complex medical management. An example of this is the case report by Otto and colleagues.[38] The case discussed teleultrasonography consultation between cardiologists at the University of Texas at Galveston and staff in a research center in Antarctica about a patient with pericarditis. The use of this technology prevented unnecessary medical evacuation and transfer, allowing the patient to receive treatment at the center. Other promising applications of tele-echocardiography have been seen on the International Space Station and in heart transplant procurement.[39,40]

ROBOTIC CARDIAC CATHETERIZATION

In the PRECISE (Percutaneous Robotically Enhanced Coronary Intervention) study, Weisz and colleagues[41] showed that robotic percutaneous coronary intervention by means of the CorPath 200 robotic system (Corindus Vascular Robotics, Waltham, MA) was successful in 98.8% of patients. The system consists of a remote interventional cockpit with a bedside disposable cassette that facilitates operator-guided manipulation of guidewires, catheters, stents, and balloons. In the current study, the operator remained in the same catheterization laboratory as the patient. Remote robotic cardiac catheterization trials are currently being formulated in which the operator will attempt revascularization from a distant site. In the future, this may enable patients from underserved regions to derive the benefit of percutaneous intervention.

CHRONIC HEART FAILURE MONITORING

There are currently more than 5 million Americans with a known diagnosis of heart failure and about 650,000 new diagnoses are made yearly.[42] An additional 3 million patients are expected to develop heart failure in the United States by 2030.[43] The worsening heart failure epidemic is a significant driver of health care expenditure. The cost of health care services, medications, and lost productivity caused by heart failure was estimated to exceed $30 billion in 2013, with the mean cost of a heart failure admission averaging about $23,000.[42] The United States Centers for Medicare and Medicaid Services began public reporting of all-cause readmission rates after a heart failure admission in 2009.[44] Subsequently, the Patient Protection and Affordable Care Act of 2010 established financial penalties for hospitals with the highest readmission rates within 30 days of discharge.[45] Thus, there is an unmet need to develop new strategies to improve heart failure care overall, and a particular focus to reduce readmissions specifically.

Notable progress in heart failure management has been made with new drug therapies and remote monitoring of patients with heart failure. Because of the labor-intensive nature of heart failure management, remote monitoring has become appealing, and is potentially a cost-effective method of home management and prevention of readmission. Telemedicine support in particular has evolved to include telephone communication or electronic monitoring with peripheral devices and video consultation.[46] Many studies have had conflicting data regarding the improved outcomes related to telemedicine in caring for patients with heart failure.

Rich and colleagues[47] showed that nursing-directed, multidisciplinary inventions, including education, and follow-up (individualized home visits and telephone contact) reduced the rates of readmission substantially and increased quality-of-life scores. A clinical trial by Riegel and colleagues[48] indicated that standardized nurse case management provided to sick patients with heart failure by telephone in the first 6 months after discharge can provided cost savings, less resource use, and improved patient satisfaction.

HEART FAILURE MONITORING

Various forms of supportive monitoring have evolved to care for the medically complex heart failure population.

Telephone-based Monitoring

One form of support is via telephone. Nursing-directed live phone calls are made to patients and information regarding patients' status is collected at intermittent periods.

If there seems to be a clinical change or progressive deterioration, patients are instructed to go to their physician or hospital for follow-up. The studies vary in design and in the level and complexity of intervention.

Riegel and colleagues[48] placed a heavy emphasis on patient education. The patients' clinical statuses were followed by registered nurses for the first 6 months after discharge. The nurses were also instructed to educate patients regarding their disease processes and to emphasize deterioration of illness with the help of decision support software. Reports of clinical statuses were sent to the patients' physicians, who in turn chose appropriate interventions and therapies. This process was able to reduce hospitalization rates by close to 50% and reduce inpatient costs. In DeBusk and colleagues'[49] study in 2004, low-risk patients with heart failure were randomized to nursing intervention with regular care or regular care alone. The intervention group received symptoms monitoring, education, and medications for heart failure with the help of a study protocol. Patients were contacted via telephone intermittently. Additional calls and coordination of care with physicians was the responsibility of the nurse. The study showed no reduction in hospitalization rates between the two groups and thus no benefit.[49] The DIAL trial compared frequent centralized telephone intervention by a nurse trained in the management of chronic heart failure with usual care.[50] The objective was to educate and monitor the patients. The focus was adherence to diet, drug treatment, fluid status, and symptoms monitoring. The nurses used software to determine the frequency of calls, and algorithms were used to adjust the diuretic dose. With this intervention, there was a significant reduction in admissions for heart failure in the intervention group (relative risk reduction, 29%; $P = .005$). A better quality of life was noted in this group (mean total score on Minnesota Living with Heart Failure questionnaire, 30.6 v 35; $P = .001$) compared with the nonintervention group. A similar trial by Dunagan and colleagues[51] randomized patients to usual care or scheduled telephone calls by nurses emphasizing self-care and guideline-based therapy as prescribed by primary physicians. The nurses screened for heart failure decompensation and could make changes in diuretic dose accordingly. The intervention patients experienced a delay to encounter (HR, 0.67; 95% CI, 0.47–0.96; $P = .29$), hospital readmission, and heart failure–specific readmission. In the first 6 months, hospital costs, hospital days, and admissions were significantly lower but this difference was not seen at 1 year. There was little impact on quality of life, functional status, or mortality.

MORTALITY AND HEART FAILURE TELECARDIOLOGY

There are many trials with new technologies for remote monitoring related to chronic heart failure, including structured telephone calls, videophone, interactive voice-response devices, and telemonitoring (**Fig. 2**).

In the subanalysis and meta-analysis by Conway and colleagues,[52] 2 of the 4 modalities, structured telephone calls and telemonitoring, were effective in reducing the risk of all-cause mortality (relative risk [RR], 0.87; 95% CI, 0.75–1.01; $P = .06$; and RR, 0.62; 95% CI, 0.50–0.77; $P<.0001$, respectively) and heart failure–related hospitalizations (RR, 0.77; 95% CI, 0.68–0.87; $P<.001$; and RR, 0.75; 95% CI, 0.3–0.91; $P = .0003$, respectively). More randomized studies need to be done to focus on effectiveness of remote monitoring in heart failure. A meta-analysis by Clark and colleagues[53] assessed whether remote monitoring for patients with chronic heart failure (structured telephone support or telemonitoring) without regular clinic or home visits improves outcomes. Remote monitoring reduced the rates of admission to hospital for chronic heart failure by 21% (95% CI, 11%–31%)

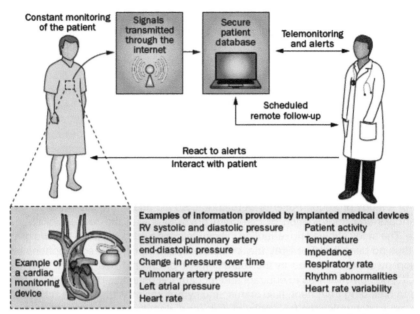

Fig. 2. Cardiac remote monitoring systems. A monitoring system in which information potentially provided from either an implantable or noninvasive device is transmitted to a secure server accessible to clinicians via the Internet. Clinicians review the data, respond to overall data trends or alerts, and communicate medical interventions directly to the patient. RV, right ventricle. (*From* Abraham WT, Stough WG, Piña IL, et al. Trials of implantable monitoring devices in heart failure: which design is optimal? Nat Rev Cardiol 2014;11(10):576–85. http://dx.doi.org/10.1038/nrcardio.2014.114; with permission.)

and all-cause mortality by 20% with benefits to quality of life and some cost benefits.

A meta-analysis by Schmidt and colleagues[54] of both telephone support and monitoring of vital signs/data concluded that scientific data on vital sign monitoring are limited, but that it may have positive effects related to mortality. Both modalities seem to be effective, but there is no evidence to suggest that one type is superior to the other.

AUTOMATED PHYSIOLOGIC MONITORING

Koehler and colleagues[55] designed a study to determine whether physician-led remote telemedical management (RTM) would reduce mortality in patients with chronic heart failure (class II or III). The system was a wireless Bluetooth device connected to an ECG monitor, a blood pressure monitor, and a weighing scale in the patients' homes. The patients performed a daily self-assessment with the devices and the data were transmitted to the telemedicine center. Physicians in the telemedicine center were available 24 hours a day, 7 days a week for consultation, instituting treatment, or in case a patient asked to speak with them. The median follow-up was 26 months. Compared with usual care, RTM had no significant effect on all-cause mortality (HR, 0.97; 95% CI, 0.67–0.41; $P = .87$) or on cardiovascular death or heart failure hospitalization. The Japanese HOMES-HF (Home Telemonitoring Study for Patients with Heart Failure) study is currently underway with the aim of investigating whether an automated physiologic monitoring system (body weight, blood pressure, pulse rate) in a heart failure treatment program could reduce mortality and readmission rates after acute decompensated heart failure.[56] All patients are New York Heart Association functional class II to III and have been discharged for the hospital within 30 days. The primary end point is a composite of all-cause death and rehospitalization because of worsening heart failure. According to the study protocol, participants were enrolled until August 2013 and followed until August 2014.

A large proportion of patients with heart failure with reduced ejection and severe left ventricular dysfunction receive device therapy in the form of implantable cardioverter defibrillators (ICDs) or cardiac resynchronization devices. It is possible to use data stored in these devices remotely to guide heart failure therapy. For example, it is possible to calculate intrathoracic impedance between pacing or ICD leads and the pulse generator. Thoracic impedance is thought to be inversely related to pulmonary fluid because water is a better conductor of electricity than air. In the FAST (Fluid Accumulation Status Trial) study intrathoracic impedance monitoring was more sensitive predictor of hospital admission for heart failure than weight measurement.[57] The However, the DOT-HF trial did not show a decrease in hospital admissions based on intrathoracic impedance monitoring and paradoxically showed an increased admission rate.[58]

Invasive monitoring of left atrial pressure by means of an investigational implantable lead sensor is currently being studied. The lead is connected to a subcutaneous antenna coil that relays left atrial pressure remotely via secure computer-based management.[59] The first observational trial using invasive left atrial pressure–guided therapy did show a decrease in heart failure admissions in patients managed with the left atrial sensor.[60] A large multicenter randomized trial, the LAPTOP-HF (Left Atrial Pressure Monitoring to Optimize Heart Failure) trial, is currently underway to validate these findings.

Despite the development of comprehensive systems for the management of patients with heart failure, hospitalization rates remain exceptionally high. In spite of systematic study of home monitoring, there is limited evidence that it improves readmission rates or mortality. Telemonitoring management has failed to show effectiveness in patients with advanced heart failure, but may show promise in low-risk patients who still require intermittent care.[61]

SUMMARY

The impact of telecardiology consultation in critically ill patients continues to evolve and includes many promising applications with potential positive implications for admission rates, morbidity, and mortality.

REFERENCES

1. Strehle EM, Shabde N. One hundred years of telemedicine: does this technology have a place in paediatrics? Arch Dis Child 2006;91(12):956–9.
2. Einthoven W. Le telecardiogramme (the telecardiogram). Arch Int Physiol 1906;4:132–64.
3. Go AS, Mozaffarian D, Roger VL, et al. Executive summary: heart disease and stroke statistics–2014 update: a report from the American Heart Association. Circulation 2014;129:399–410.
4. Morrow DA, Fang JC, Fintel DJ, et al. Evolution of critical care cardiology: transformation of the cardiovascular intensive care unit and the emerging need for

new medical staffing and training models: a scientific statement from the American Heart Association. Circulation 2012;126:1408–28.

5. Lilly CM, Cody S, Zhao H, et al. Hospital mortality, length of stay and preventable complications among critically ill patients before and after tele-ICU reengineering of critical care processes. JAMA 2011;305(21):2175–83.

6. Sadaka F, Palagiri A, Trottier S, et al. Telemedicine intervention improves ICU outcomes. Crit Care Res Pract 2013;2013:456389.

7. Nikus K, Lahteenmaki J, Lehto P, et al. The role of continuous monitoring in a 24/7 telecardiology consultation service – a feasibility study. J Electrocardiol 2009; 42(6):473–80.

8. Keeley EC, Boura JA, Grines CL. Primary angioplasty versus intravenous thrombolytic therapy for acute myocardial infarction: a quantitative review of 23 randomised trials. Lancet 2003;361:13–20.

9. Dalby M, Bouzamondo A, Lechat P, et al. Transfer for primary angioplasty versus immediate thrombolysis in acute myocardial infarction: a meta-analysis. Circulation 2003;108:1809–14.

10. O'Gara PT, Kushner FG, Ascheim DD, et al. 2013 ACCF/AHA guideline for the management of ST-elevation myocardial infarction: a report of the American College of Cardiology Foundation/American Heart Association Task Force on Practice Guidelines. Circulation 2013;127:e362–425.

11. Danchin A, Durand E, Blanchard D. Pre-hospital thrombolysis in perspective. Eur Heart J 2008;29(23):2835–42.

12. Danchin N, Blanchard P, Steg PG, et al. Impact of prehospital thrombolysis for acute myocardial infarction on 1 year outcome: results from the French Nationwide USIC 2000 registry. Circulation 2004;110(14):1909–15.

13. McLean S, Wild S, Connor P, et al. Treating ST elevation myocardial infarction by primary percutaneous coronary intervention, in-hospital thrombolysis and prehospital thrombolysis. An observational study of timelines and outcomes in 625 patients. Emerg Med J 2011;28(3):230–6.

14. Correa BS, Goncalves B, Teixeira IM, et al. AToMS: a ubiquitous teleconsultation system for supporting AMI patients with prehospital thrombolysis. Int J Telemed Appl 2011;2011:560209.

15. Bilgi M, Erol T, Gullu H, et al. Teleconsultation of coronary angiograms using smartphones and an audio/video conferencing application. Technol Health Care 2013;21(4):407–14.

16. Yousef J, Lars A. Validation of a real-time wireless telemedicine system, using bluetooth protocol and mobile phone, for remote monitoring patient in medical practice. Eur J Med Res 2005;10:254–62.

17. Giannakakis G, Buliev I. ECG signal recording, processing and transmission using a mobile phone. In: Proceedings of the 1st international conference on pervasive technologies related to assistive environments, Athens, Greece. 15–19 July 2008. New York: ACM Digital Library; 2008.

18. Hsieh J, Li A, Yang C. Mobile, cloud, and big data computing: contributions, challenges, and new directions in telecardiology. Int J Environ Res Public Health 2013;10:6131–53.

19. Chu Y, Ganz A. A mobile teletrauma system using 3G networks. IEEE Trans Inf Technol Biomed 2004;8:456–62.

20. Brunetti ND, Di Pietro G, Aquilino A, et al. Pre-hospital electrocardiogram triage with tele-cardiology support is associated with shorter time-to-balloon and higher rates of timely reperfusion even in rural areas: data from the Bari-Barletta/Andria/Trani public emergency medical service 118 registry on primary angioplasty in

ST-elevation myocardial infarction. Eur Heart J Acute Cardiovasc Care 2014;3(3): 204–13.

21. Hutchison AW, Malaiapan Y, Jarvie I, et al. Prehospital and emergency department activation of the infarct team significantly improves door-to-door times: ambulance Victoria and MonashHEART Acute Myocardial Infarction (MonAMI) 12-lead ECG project. Circ Cardiovasc Interv 2009;2:528–34.

22. Rasmussen MB, Frost L, Stengaard C, et al. Diagnostic performance and system delay using telemedicine for prehospital diagnosis in triage and treatment of STEMI. Heart 2014;100(9):711–5.

23. Sivagangabalan G, Ong AT, Narayan A, et al. Effect of prehospital triage on revascularization times, left ventricular function, and survival in patients with ST-elevation myocardial infarction. Am J Cardiol 2009;103(7):907–12.

24. Chan AW, Kornder J, Elliott H, et al. Improved survival associated with prehospital strategy in a large regional ST-segment elevation myocardial infarction program. JACC Cardiovasc Interv 2012;5(12):1239–46.

25. McCabe JM, Armstrong EJ, Ku I, et al. Physician accuracy in interpreting potential ST-segment elevation myocardial infarction electrocardiograms. J Am Heart Assoc 2013;2(5):e000268.

26. Brunetti ND, Dellegrottaglie G, Lopriore C, et al. Prehospital telemedicine electrocardiogram triage for a regional public emergency medical service: is it worth it? A preliminary cost analysis. Clin Cardiol 2014;37(3):140–5.

27. Finley JP, Sharratt GP, Nanton MA, et al. Paediatric echocardiography by telemedicine—nine years' experience. J Telemed Telecare 1997;3(4):200–4.

28. Trippi JA, Lee KS, Kopp G, et al. Emergency echocardiography telemedicine: an efficient method to provide 24-hour consultative echocardiography. J Am Coll Cardiol 1996;27:1748–52.

29. Trippi JA, Kopp A, Lee KS, et al. The feasibility of dobutamine stress echocardiography in the emergency department with telemedicine interpretation. J Am Soc Echocardiogr 1996;9(2):113–8.

30. Trippi JA, Lee KS, Kopp G, et al. Dobutamine stress tele-cardiography for evaluation of emergency department patients with chest pain. J Am Coll Cardiol 1997;30:627–32.

31. Prinz C, Dohrmann J, Buuren FV, et al. Diagnostic performance of handheld echocardiography for the assessment of basic cardiac morphology and function: a validation study in routine cardiac patients. Echocardiography 2012;29(8): 887–94.

32. Choi BG, Mukherjee M, Dala P, et al. Interpretation of remotely downloaded pocket-sized cardiac ultrasound images on a web-enabled smartphone: validation against workstation evaluation. J Am Soc Echocardiogr 2011;24:1325–30.

33. Grant B, Morgan GJ, McCrossan BA, et al. Remote diagnosis of congenital heart disease: the impact of telemedicine. Arch Dis Child 2010;95:270–80.

34. Dowie R, Mistry H, Yound TA, et al. Cost implications of introducing a telecardiology service to support fetal ultrasound screening. J Telemed Telecare 2008;14:412–22.

35. Haley JE, Klewer SE, Barber BJ, et al. Remote diagnosis of congenital heart disease in southern Arizona: comparison between tele-cardiography and videotapes. Telemed J E Health 2012;18(10):736–42.

36. Courreges F, Vieyres P, Istepanian R, et al. Clinical trials and evaluation of a mobile, robotic tele-ultrasound system. J Telemed Telecare 2005;11(Suppl 1): 46–9.

37. Available at: http://www.itnonline.com/article/statvideos-echocart-streams-tele-echocardiography-images-babies'-hearts-duke-childrens-hospi. Accessed October 10, 2014.

38. Otto CA, Shemenski R, Drudi L. Real-time tele-echocardiography: diagnosis and management of a pericardial effusion secondary to pericarditis at an Antarctic research station. Telemed J E Health 2012;18(7):521–4.
39. Hamilton DR, Sargsyyan AE, Martin DS, et al. On-orbit prospective echocardiography on International Space Station crew. Echocardiography 2011;28(5):491–501.
40. Franchi D, Davide C, Arpesella G, et al. Second-opinion stress tele-echocardiography for the Adonhers (Aged donor heart rescue by stress echo) project. Cardiovasc Ultrasound 2010;8:20.
41. Weisz G, Metzger DC, Caputo RP, et al. Safety and feasibility of robotic percutaneous coronary intervention: PRECISE (percutaneous robotically-enhanced coronary intervention) study. J Am Coll Cardiol 2013;61:1596–600.
42. Yancy CW, Jessup M, Bozkurt B, et al. 2013 ACCF/AHA guideline for the management of heart failure: a report of the American College of Cardiology Foundation/American Heart Association Task Force on Practice Guidelines. J Am Coll Cardiol 2013;62:e147–239.
43. Vigen R, Maddox TM, Allen LA. Aging of the United States population: impact on heart failure. Curr Heart Fail Rep 2012;9:369–74.
44. Desai AS, Stevenson LW. Rehospitalization for heart failure: predict or prevent? Circulation 2012;126:501–6.
45. Available at: http://housedocs.house.gov/energycommerce/ppacacon.pdf. Accessed October 10, 2014.
46. Riley JP, Cowie MR. Telemonitoring in heart failure. Heart 2009;95:1964–8.
47. Rich MW, Beckham V, Wittenberg C, et al. A multidisciplinary intervention to prevent the readmission of elderly patients with congestive heart failure. N Engl J Med 1995;333:1190–5.
48. Riegel B, Carlson B, Kopp Z, et al. Effect of a standardized nurse case-management telephone intervention on resource use in patients with chronic heart failure. Arch Intern Med 2002;162(6):705–12.
49. DeBusk RF, Miller NH, Parker KM, et al. Care management for low-risk patients with heart failure, a randomized, control trial. Ann Intern Med 2004;141:606–13.
50. GESICA Investigators. Randomised trial of telephone intervention in chronic heart failure: DIAL trial. BMJ 2005;331:425.
51. Dunagan WC, Littenberg B, Ewald GA, et al. Randomized trial of a nurse-administered, telephone-based disease management for patients with heart failure. J Card Fail 2005;11(5):358–65.
52. Conway A, Inglis SC, Clark RA. Effective technologies for noninvasive remote monitoring in heart failure. Telemed J E Health 2014;20(6):531–8.
53. Clark RA, Inglis SC, McAlister FA, et al. Telemonitoring or structured telephone support programmes for patients with chronic heart failure: systemic review and meta-analysis. BMJ 2007;334:942.
54. Schmidt S, Schuchert A, Krieg T, et al. Home telemonitoring in patients with chronic heart failure. Dtsch Arztebl Int 2010;107(8):131–8.
55. Koehler F, Winkler S, Scheiber M, et al. Impact of remote telemedicine management on mortality and hospitalizations in ambulatory patients with chronic heart failure. Circulation 2011;123:1873–80.
56. Kotooka N, Asaka M, Sato Y, et al. Home Telemonitoring Study for Japanese Patients with Heart Failure (HOMES-HF): protocol for a multicenter randomized controlled trial. BMJ Open 2013;3(6):e002972.
57. Abraham WT, Compton S, Haas G, et al. Intrathoracic impedance vs daily weight monitoring for predicting worsening heart failure events: results of the Fluid Accumulation Status Trial (FAST). Congest Heart Fail 2011;17:51–5.

58. van Veldhuisen DJ, Braunschweig F, Conraads V, et al. Intrathoracic impedance monitoring, audible patient alerts, and outcome in patients with heart failure. Circulation 2011;124:1719–26.

59. Abraham WT. Remote heart failure monitoring. Curr Treat Options Cardiovasc Med 2013;15:556–64.

60. Ritzema J, Troughton R, Melton I, et al. Physician-directed patient self-management of left atrial pressure in advanced chronic heart failure. Circulation 2010;121:1086–95.

61. Hernandex AF, Greiner MA, Fonarow GC, et al. Relationship between early physician follow-up and 30-day readmission among Medicare beneficiaries hospitalized for heart failure. JAMA 2010;303:1716–22.

Practice Challenges of Intensive Care Unit Telemedicine

Herb Rogove, DO[a],*, Kory Stetina, CPC[b]

KEYWORDS

- TeleICU • Telemedicine • Telehealth • Medical license portability • Reimbursement
- Telemedicine credentialing • Billing • Coding

KEY POINTS

- Understanding the key challenges that face the practice of telemedicine and how that impedes the spread of technology for the benefit of telemedicine-provided patient care.
- Why state medical licensure has remained a key barrier for the adaption of telemedicine for many years.
- How hospital staff credentialing is a time-consuming activity that could easily be simplified by credentialing-by-proxy and other process improvements.
- Medicare, Medicaid, and private insurance guidelines for telehealth reimbursement can be easily accessed and analyzed, and in many cases demonstrate available reimbursement for Tele-ICU programs.
- Understanding telehealth reimbursement guidelines and the appropriate billing codes for the Tele-ICU program can empower providers to develop detailed financial projections for Tele-ICU services.

INTRODUCTION

The practice of intensive care unit (ICU) telemedicine or Tele-ICU has been available for approximately 20 years. A recently published lexicon described the types of Tele-ICUs that exist, ranging from a centralized model to a de-centralized model; open, closed, or hybrid architecture; fixed or portable technology; and care models that range from continuous, scheduled, or reactive.[1] Regardless of the model that is adapted by a hospital or health system, there are significant impediments in starting and maintaining a Tele-ICU practice. In a survey of acute-care practitioners using telemedicine, it was noted that procurement of state medical licenses, credentialing, and reimbursement

Disclosures: None.
[a] C3O Telemedicine, 1119 North Signal Street, Ojai, CA 93023, USA; [b] Torch Health Solutions, 4740 32nd Street, San Diego, CA 92116, USA
* Corresponding author.
E-mail address: herb.rogove@c3otelemedicine.com

Crit Care Clin 31 (2015) 319–334
http://dx.doi.org/10.1016/j.ccc.2014.12.009
0749-0704/15/$ – see front matter © 2015 Elsevier Inc. All rights reserved.

criticalcare.theclinics.com

were major barriers to telemedicine.[2] This article presents the historic developments in the context of proposed solutions with an understanding of the difficulties to achieve a more uniform and easy process to rapidly advance the field of telemedicine.

STATE MEDICAL LICENSURE

There are currently 70 state medical boards in the United States. As required for on-site medical practice, telemedicine is not exempt from obtaining either a full license or a special license to practice in each of the 50 states and territories. Each state issues its own statutes as to how medicine will be practiced, and this is accomplished through each of the state medical boards. Additionally, some states have added special requirements, such as Texas, which has a jurisprudence test, Kentucky has an HIV test, and Mississippi has an on-site open-book test and video to be watched that can be done only in Jackson, Mississippi. The licensing system in the United States has been in existence for more than a century and creates requirements that lack uniformity among all the states. The creation of this model is based on the policing responsibilities of each state, including that for the medical profession. As a result, the state medical boards have taken their responsibility to protect the safety of their citizens as the core mission of how the medical boards regulate the issuance of a license to practice medicine. Unfortunately, with the development of technology such as telemedicine, medical licensure has not adapted to the 21st century and as a result the practice of medicine through telemedicine and across state boundaries has produced a conundrum for health care systems and telemedicine companies in this growing field of medical practice. The citizens of each state, particularly those who live in medically underserved areas, are the ones most often affected by these state regulations and often are required to travel hundreds of miles to seek needed care.

The Beginning: Government and Grants

Interest in telemedicine by both the federal and state governments dates back to the 1990s. In fact, by 1994 there were 18 federal agencies involved in telemedicine, with a budget of $85 million for program development.[3] In 1995, then congressional representative Ron Wyden (D-OR), who is one of the current senators representing Oregon, proposed an amendment to the Communications Act of 1995 to prevent states from restricting interstate telemedicine consultations.[4] This bill was ultimately withdrawn.

The Federation of State Medical Boards (FSMB) has been at the center of many of the nongovernment agencies trying to address the licensure portability issue for years. In 1996, the FSMB adopted a Model Act, which called on state medical boards to adopt a "special-purpose license" to issue limited practice for telemedicine in states beyond where the physician held a current license.[5] The Model Act was adopted by only 8 states.

One year later in 1997, the Office of the Department of Commerce and the Office for the Advancement of Telehealth (OAT), which is a part of the Department of Health and Human Services (HHS), issued a report to Congress identifying licensure as a barrier for telemedicine. Again in 2001, the OAT updated the 1997 report stating again that licensure remains a major barrier to the development of telemedicine.[6]

At about the same time, the National Council of State Boards of Nursing approved a Nurse Licensure Compact in 1998 in which states could agree to recognize a license granted by another participating state. Unfortunately, only 23 states currently have adopted the compact over the course of 16 years.[7]

The FSMB continued to provide leadership, first by establishing, in 2000, a special committee on licensure portability.[5] In 2002, the House Commerce Committee added language to the Safety Net legislation, section 102, expressing interest in collaboration among regulatory boards to facilitate the elimination of barriers to telehealth practice.[5] In this legislation, grants were offered to state medical boards to promote cooperation and to encourage the development and introduction of state laws to reduce the statutory and regulatory barriers for telemedicine licensing.[6]

Then, in 2004 and 2005 the OAT requested a model interstate agreement to facilitate licensure portability across state lines. In 2006, the first grant FSMB received from the OAT produced the Common Licensure Application Form (CLAF) working in conjunction with Federation Certification Verification Service of the FSMB. The goal was for state medical boards to scan and share licensure documents in electronic formats.[6] Then in 2009, the second grant produced the Uniform Application (UA), which was an update to CLAF, and expedited endorsement agreements.[6] In 2006, Congress appropriated funds by creating the Licensure Portability Grant Program.[6] The FSMB received funds from this grant as well. One year prior, in 2005, the OAT also engaged the FSMB to help on this same issue.

Although Congress and the FSMB had been working for a solution, state leadership at the governor's level began discussions. This included the Midwest Governors Association, Western Governors Association, Southern Governors Association (SGA), Coalition of Northeastern Governors, Council on Great Lakes Governors, and the New England Governors Conference.[8] This appeared at first glance as an excellent breakthrough, as state leaders were discussing the telemedicine licensure barrier and all knew the need to leverage telemedicine for their own rural hospitals and clinics. On a state level, the National Governors Association created the State Alliance for E-Health.[5] In 1999, the SGA formed the Task Force on Medical Technology and issued a report "From Promise to Practice—Improving Life in the South through Telemedicine."[8] In that same year, Alabama, Tennessee, and Texas adapted the FSMB model for reciprocity. Unfortunately, none of these endeavors seemed to impact most state medical boards to change their practice of accepting other state's medical license.

In 2010, a Health Resources and Services Administration (HRSA) Report was issued known as Senate Report 111-66, which had been requested by the Departments of Labor, HHS, and Education and related agencies.[5] The intent of the report was to provide an update on the licensure portability. Essentially the report summarized what had already been described, which was that each state created variable barriers to securing a medical license. In that same year, 2010, HRSA awarded the FSMB another grant from funds from the American Recovery and Reinvestment Act of 2009 P.L. 111-5 Licensure portability.[6] The report mentioned the FSMB's encouragement of states to accept expedited endorsement. At that time, 8 states, which included Idaho, Michigan, Nevada, New Mexico, North Carolina, Oregon, and Rhode Island, adapted expedited endorsement. Widespread state adoption never occurred.

It can be concluded that many at both the state and federal levels have studied and made suggestions for an immediate change to the process of the attainment of a multistate medical license; however, a consensus by all the medical boards never emerged (**Box 1**).

Prominent Federal Telehealth Legislation

The past 10 years and in particular the past 3 years have seen state and federal legislators both understand and then introduce legislation that recognizes the importance of telemedicine for the present and the future (**Box 2**). Although many state medical boards fear loss of state authority, one only needs to understand that physicians have the ability to legally practice anywhere in the 25-nation European Union. Australia has already moved away from a state-based system to a single national agency that

---

Box 1
Historic timeline

1996 FSMB Model Act

   HHS and Department of Commerce report to Congress

1997 Congressional Report: OAT

1998 Nursing Compact

2001 Congressional Report: OAT

   FSMB updates 1996 report

2002 Safety Net legislation

2004-05 OAT contract to FSMB

2006 OAT grant to FSMB

2007 ATA issues policy

2008 ABA Health Law section issues a model

   State Alliance for E-Health issues a report

2009 Consensus statements from 22 State medical boards, ONC, HSS, National Governors Association, FSMB

   Second OAT grant to FSMB

2010 HRSA grant to FSMB

   FCC Plan

2014 FSMB Interstate Compact – revision July, 2014

Abbreviations: ABA, American Bar Association; ATA, American Telemedicine Association; FCC, Federal Communications Commission; FSMB, Federation of State Medical Boards; HHS, Department of Health and Human Services; OAT, Office for the Advancement of Telehealth (part of HRSA); ONC, Office of National Coordinator.

---

administrates a regulation and accreditation program for all physicians.[9] Therefore, to keep the United States on a similar path to adapt to the 21st century, our nation needs to see by example what the rest of the world is doing to embrace new technologies to enhance patient care. Second, no one is asking for the states to surrender their right to discipline and monitor physicians who have not upheld the medical board's standards of safe practice.

Box 2
Prominent legislation for telemedicine license portability

2004 Senate Bill 2325, Telehealth Improvement Act of 2004

2011 HR 1832: Servicemembers' Telemedicine and E-Health Portability Act of 2011 (STEP Act)

2013 HR 2001: Veterans E-Health and Telemedicine Support Act of 2013

2013 HR 3077: TELE-MED Act of 2013

2013 HR 3750: Telehealth Modernization Act of 2013

2013 HR 3306: Telehealth Enhancement Act of 2013

2014 HR 5380: Medicare Telehealth Parity Act; S.2662: Telehealth Enhancement Act

Focusing specifically on federal legislation, one of the earliest bills introduced in the past 10 years was the Telehealth Improvement Act of 2004, known as Senate Bill 2325, introduced by Senator John Edwards (D-NC) requiring the Secretary of HHS to convene a conference of state licensing boards, local telehealth projects, health care practitioners, and patient advocates to promote interstate licensure for telehealth projects.[10] This bill never progressed and ultimately died.

On May 11, 2011, Representative Glenn Thompson (R-PA5) introduced the Service-members' Telemedicine and E-Health Portability Act of 2011 (also known as the STEP Act), which authorized the Secretary of Defense (Department of Defense [DOD]) to allow certain licensed health care professionals to provide care to members of the Armed Forces from anywhere the health care professional or the patient was located. The one caveat was that the practice was within the scope of authorized federal duty. With this Act, even civilians, DOD employees, or contractors were eligible if they were credentialed and privileged at federal health care facilities.[11] To monitor this initiative, the Secretary of Defense was to provide Congress with a report on the program and how it affects patient access and program development.

Representative Charles Rangel (D-NY13) introduced on May 15, 2013, HR 2001: Veterans E-Health & Telemedicine Support Act of 2013. This legislation allows a health care professional who is authorized to provide health care through the Department of Veterans Affairs (VA) and who is a licensed professional to practice at any location in any state, the District of Columbia, or a US commonwealth, territory, or possession, regardless of where the professional or patient is located, if the professional is using telemedicine to provide treatment. The bill allows such treatment regardless of whether such professional or patient is located in a facility owned by the federal government.[12] So far, discussion at the VA Subcommittee on Health has yet to progress.

One of the key legislations regarding licensure portability was contained in the TELE-MED Act of 2013, introduced as HR 3077 by Representative Devin Nunes (R-CA 22) on September 10, 2013, to permit certain Medicare providers licensed in one state to provide telemedicine services to a Medicare beneficiary in a different state.[13] No action has been taken at the time of publication.

On October 22, 2013, The Telehealth Enhancement Act of 2013, known as HR 3306, was introduced by Representative Greg Harper (R-MS3) to expand the role of telehealth in preventing hospital readmissions, encourage the medical home, include telehealth in Accountable Care Organizations and require the Federal Communications Commission (FCC) to develop rules that will enhance provider access to patient information and services regardless of provider location.[14]

Representative Doris Matsui (D-CA6) introduced the Telehealth Modernization Act of 2013, known as HR 3750, on December 12, 2013, seeking to codify the definition of "telehealth" at the federal level to promote participation and acceptance of remote care.[15] The bill would establish guidelines for states to improve their telehealth capabilities and recommend new licensing laws.

Companion bills introduced in both the House and the Senate occurred on July 31 and July 24, 2014, respectively. The Senate version, The Telehealth Enhancement Act (S 2262) was introduced by Senators Thad Cochran (R-MS) and Roger Wicker (R-MS) and addresses store-and-forward, home care, expansion of telemedicine coverage to Metropolitan Statistical Areas (MSAs), and expansion of types of health care providers and diagnoses. Congressman Mike Thompson (D-CA) introduced the congressional companion bill, Medicare Telehealth Parity Act, HR 5380, which is a 3-phase bill analogous to S 2262.[16,17]

Despite some encouraging legislation that displays a keen sense of understanding both the problem that was being solved and patient need, none of these bills to date have shown any signs of accelerated adoption or proceeding out of committee for a vote, despite having bipartisan support.

Uniformity: Legal Exploration—Interstate Commerce

During the past 10 years, conversations were beginning to emerge as some felt that telemedicine, in legal terms, is a form of interstate commerce. This was an attempt to pave the way for a federal mandate. Discussions concentrated around a federally issued license or even a national license. Advocates claimed that in this scenario the 10th amendment of the US Constitution might not be absolute for the states because of the Commerce Clause.[8] What this means is that the 10th amendment gave power to the states for certain areas rather than the federal government. Such a power was for the states to establish how to license physicians. This was challenged by some attorneys based on the Commerce Clause, which gives the right to Congress, not an individual state, to control interstate commerce, of which the delivery of medical care is being argued as qualifying as interstate commerce. However, a large movement toward this end never emerged, in part because of the complexity of setting up another agency to oversee the program and of course the costs associated with such an agency.

Another legal idea emerged by reviewing the efforts of the National Conference of Commissioners of Uniform State Law adapted by 49 states to maintain a general uniformity of state law.[5] This august body was made up of attorneys, judges, and legislators. Applying this concept to medical licensure also failed to gain enough support to move telemedicine licensure portability on parity of state law for medical licenses to have uniformity from state to state.

A third argument emerged in favor of a national or federal license. The precedent was based on the Mammography Quality Standards Act of 1992. Here Congress passed this law allowing the Food and Drug Administration to establish national standards for mammography facilities and their staff.[5]

Finally, back in 1973, the federal government established the Health Maintenance Organization law, which preempted state laws against the corporate practice of medicine.[18] Although there appears to be legal precedent, the politics of the day appeared to favor the state right to maintain its law as usual and to accommodate new technology and a changing world. Again, this approach never gained a stronghold.

Professional Organizations Join the Cause

Professional organizations support ideas and solutions, which had begun in 1996. In 2011, the American Telemedicine Association (ATA), the leading advocacy group for telemedicine, issued a policy encouraging resolution of this major problem, as now many companies and physician service organizations that wanted to provide telehealth consultation to some of the most needed areas of our country were being thwarted by antiquated regulations and large expenses.[19]

In 2008, the American Bar Association's Health Law Section issued a statement requesting legislators and regulators to change their old laws to meet the new practice needs of telemedicine. They said "the most significant restraints on the full growth of telemedicine in the United States and the rest of the world are the legal barriers that remain—and are still being created."[20]

Also, in 2008, the State Alliance for E-Health, a special committee of the National Governors Association issued a statement requesting the state medical boards to institute a system of mutual licensure recognition. This concept of reciprocity by which each state recognizes another state's license is a very simple process that the states can do on their own, thereby simplifying the process immensely. The statement also recognized that the physician pay the appropriate fees, be subject to discipline, and adhere to the state's professional standards of care.[20]

In 2010, the FCC suggested that the nation's governors and state legislators collaborate in conjunction with the National Governors Association and the FSMB. In that statement, the group was given 18 months to come up with a plan or Congress would intervene. The 18 months had passed and no new legislation from this organization followed nor did the federal government intervene.[6]

Most recently, the ATA in 2013 started the Fix Licensure program advocating for a rapid fix for an archaic licensing system. On that site, the ATA comments "The current approach, requiring health providers to obtain multiple state licenses and adhere to diverse and sometimes conflicting state medical practice rules, is a barrier to progress, quality, competition and economy. This partitioned approach also presents a concern for patient safety as state-by-state licensing and enforcement inhibits tracking down and disciplining bad doctors located in other states."[21]

Licensure Models

Sorting out all of the attempts at both state and federal legislation, several licensure models have been proposed as solutions to the portability issue. Included in the discussion has been the desire to have a UA, and to that end it has been created but a major drawback has been that not all states accept it nor do they allow electronic submission. However, the overarching impediment is to have a model that allows for the most painless and efficient means to practice in multiple states. The following are the more commonly discussed models.[6]

- Full Licensure: physician must apply for a license in each state.
- Mutual Recognition: states recognize and accept other state's license. This could be in the form of a compact or other means as determined by the states.
- Limited or Special-Purpose License: proposed by FSMB in 2000 in which the state grants access only to telemedicine and the physician cannot physically practice in that state. The physician must also abide by regulatory controls of the state in which the patient resides.
- Endorsement: the state with equivalent standards accepts the license but may require additional regulations to be completed.
- Expedited (FSMB Compact): physician files with his or her home state and the other state(s) decides to verify with no primary source verification needed. If approved, the physician then fills out an application and pays the fee to the new state.
- Reciprocity: states need to negotiate an agreement to accept each other state's medical license.
- Registration: the physician only needs to register.
- Consulting Exceptions: at the request and in consultation with an on-site physician. This has been discussed even before telehealth arrived and is of limited value to the current discussion.
- National License: based on a universal standard for practice in the United States.
- Federal License: federally issued and standards are federal but states might play a role in implementation.

Where Are We Now?

In late April of 2014, and revised in July 2014, the FSMB met to discuss licensure portability. The Interstate Medical Licensure Compact was presented and subsequently passed. In the Interstate Medical Licensure Compact, a physician in the home state would apply to his or her home state's medical board, which would verify or deny the applicant's eligibility. Once the application is verified, the physician does not need to have any additional primary verification, which would cut the process time substantially. After verification from the home state and a fee to the new state(s), the requested state(s) will then issue a medical license. A Commission made up of a representative from each state's medical board would establish the administration of this Interstate Medical License Compact.[22]

It is important to keep in mind that the FSMB Compact essentially provides for an expedited license. This means that physicians are still required to have full licensure issued by each and every state but now with an expedited application process. One might argue that the easiest process would be for states to simply accept another state's medical license as proof of competency, analogous to how a driver's license is accepted by all states.

As far as legislation, we are still waiting to see if any of the previously discussed congressional resolutions will make it out of committee. Understanding how these same regulations can apply to nongovernment hospitals will be another challenge.

Next Steps

So what can goal-driven intensivists who wish to practice ICU telemedicine do? As what has been discussed, it is evident that the evolutionary process of securing an easy medical license across home state borders is time-consuming, costly, and extremely frustrating. The cost to physicians alone amounts to more than $300 million a year (Jonathan Linkous, CEO, ATA, personal communication, 2014). In fact, if one would go to the federation of state medical board licensure Web site (http://www.fsmb.org/) and calculate the cost to obtain licenses in all 50 states, the grand total would be about $24,118. It appears that active involvement in organizations such as the ATA is one way to be informed and have input, as the ATA has a full-time director of public policy who is intimately involved in activities on Capitol Hill. Establishing communication with your congressional representative and senator is also important. Because several resolutions have been introduced, asking your representative to support or cosponsor legislation is extremely valuable and requires only an e-mail or telephone call. Connecting with the FSMB and, more importantly, with the members of your state medical board, to share your understanding and opinion that a better process for medical license portability is essential. More needs to be done in this changing world of technology and the crisis of medical care access for our patients. A strong talking point is the anticipated shortage of intensivists that has already been publically acknowledged as a crisis with little hope for an immediate solution for more bedside intensivists.

CREDENTIALING AND PRIVILEGING

There are 2 stages a practitioner must complete to practice medicine at a hospital. The first, credentialing, is for the hospital to evaluate and verify the qualifications of the practitioner. Each hospital determines individually the qualifications. In fact, hospitals within the same health care system may have different qualifications and lack an easy and standardized process.

During the credentialing process, a second stage, the privileging, also must occur. The privileging is for the verification of the physician's competency in his or her particular specialty. Needless to say, these processes add significant time and expense to this process. This is only compounded by the lack of standardization. Now, in addition to obtaining state licenses, the added procedure of credentialing and privileging for medical groups, health care systems, or companies engaged in telemedicine is an enormous burden that only prolongs the process of providing care to patients in need.

For a time, beginning in 2004, hospitals that lacked certain specialists were able to do "credentialing-by-proxy," which was approved by The Joint Commission (TJC) but not the Centers for Medicare and Medicaid Services (CMS) (Jonathan Linkous, CEO, ATA, personal communication, 2014). The main reason the CMS could not accept the proxy was that it was in conflict with the definition of Medicare Conditions of Participation (CoP). Hospitals that took care of Medicare and Medicaid patients were required to be compliant with CoPs.[23]

The hospital receiving care, called the originating site, by the specialist was given credentials based on the acceptance of the credentials provided by the distant site (where the specialist was located). As a result, duplication and cost were greatly reduced. This worked well for financially challenged smaller and rural hospitals. It is important to point out that the practice of telemedicine required the same regulation as on-site care. This keystone decision has been advocated for all aspects of practicing, whether it is by telemedicine or on-site care is that the standards should be the same. Ultimately, the hospital's decision to use credentialing-by-proxy is totally voluntary.

It was not until July 2011, after multiple hearings and public support, that CMS finally accepted the TJC criteria for credentialing-by-proxy.[24] The criteria included the following (**Box 3**):

(1) A written agreement between the 2 parties, (2) the distant-site hospital is a Medicare-participating hospital or telemedicine entity, (3) the telehealth provider is privileged at the distant-site hospital, (4) a current list of the telehealth provider's privileges is given to the originating-site hospital, (5) the telehealth provider holds a license issued or is recognized by the state in which the originating-site hospital is located, (6) the originating-site hospital has an internal review of the telehealth provider's performance and provides this information to the distant-site hospital, (7) the originating-site hospital must inform the distant-site hospital of all adverse events, and (8) complaints regarding the services provided by the telehealth provider.

A "telemedicine entity" is defined as follows: providing telemedicine services, is not a Medicare-participating hospital, and provides its services in a manner that allows the originating-site hospital or the Critical Access Hospital (CAH) to comply with all applicable CoPs and standards.[24]

Box 3
Credentialing-by-proxy requirements

1. A written agreement between the 2 parties.

2. The distant-site hospital is a Medicare-participating hospital or telemedicine entity.

3. The telehealth provider is privileged at the distant-site hospital.

4. A current list of the telehealth provider's privileges is given to the originating-site hospital.

5. The telehealth provider holds a license issued or is recognized by the state in which the originating-site hospital is located.

6. The originating-site hospital has an internal review of the telehealth provider's performance and provides this information to the distant-site hospital.

7. The originating-site hospital must inform the distant-site hospital of all adverse events.

8. Complaints regarding the services provided by the telehealth provider.

Additionally, "If the distant site is a telemedicine entity, it must be in the written agreement that it is furnishing its services in a manner that allows the originating-site hospital or the CAH to comply with all applicable CoPs and standards. The originating-site hospital must ensure that the services provided comply with all applicable CoPs and standards."[24]

The success of having TJC and the CMS agree is attributed to the work done by many individuals, legislators, and organizations, such as the ATA and the Center for Telehealth and eHealth Law, resulting in this regulation being passed. However, although credentialing-by-proxy has been in effect since 2011, there are still hospitals that do not use it.

REIMBURSEMENT

Lack of available reimbursement for Tele-ICU physician services is thought to be a long-standing barrier to the rapid adoption of Tele-ICU programs.[25] Despite this perception, there have been a number of recent regulatory and legislative changes expanding reimbursement for telehealth services, as well as a series of recent publications and reports, all of which can assist in determining just how significant the reimbursement barrier really is for Tele-ICU providers.

The purpose of this section is to review the reimbursement guidelines for telehealth services across 3 major patient insurance classes: Medicare, Medicaid, and private insurance. After understanding which payers reimburse for telehealth services, a model will be proposed to assist new or existing Tele-ICU programs in creating financial projections to determine exactly what reimbursement is available, if any, for the Tele-ICU program.

Summary of Financial Classes

The 3 major financial classes, or patient insurance types, that will be reviewed for purposes of this analysis will be Medicare, Medicaid, and private insurance.

Medicare is a federally organized program, and its guidelines for telehealth reimbursement are generally consistent across the country, regardless of state.[26] Although guidelines are consistent across the country with few exceptions, the actual Medicare Physician Fee Schedule amounts are adjusted by geographic locality to adjust for a variation in practice costs.[27] Although physician or facility payment amounts may differ slightly by geographic region, Tele-ICU providers can determine available reimbursement by reviewing the federal guidelines for telehealth reimbursement, which are summarized later in this article.

Although state Medicaid program guidelines for telehealth reimbursement must conform to federal requirements of efficiency, economy, and quality of care, states are given flexibility to develop individual policies for telehealth reimbursement.[28] Therefore, understanding Tele-ICU reimbursement policies within state Medicaid programs requires analysis of each state's individual telehealth reimbursement guidelines. A series of reports have been published recently that find that state Medicaid program policies can vary significantly by state.[29]

Similar to Medicaid, telehealth reimbursement by private insurance companies is also determined at the state level and therefore each state's regulation of private insurance reimbursement, or lack thereof, will impact a Tele-ICU program's ability to obtain reimbursement from this financial class.[30]

Medicare

The Medicare Learning Network publishes an annual document that aims to summarize the Medicare program's guidelines for telehealth reimbursement.[26] This summary document separates the various requirements a program must meet to obtain reimbursement, including the following:

1. Originating sites (or eligible health facilities)
2. Distant-site practitioners (or eligible provider types)
3. Telehealth services (or eligible services)
4. Billing and payment for professional services furnished via telehealth
5. Billing and payment for the originating-site facility fee
6. Resources and lists of other applicable information

Although most Tele-ICU programs can meet many of the eligibility requirements described in these guidelines, the most significant requirements for determining eligible reimbursement from Medicare for Tele-ICU programs are related to the guidelines assigned to originating sites and telehealth services.

Currently, Medicare restricts any form of payment for telehealth services only to services that are provided to a patient in a facility located in a rural area. Medicare defines this restriction by requiring the facility to be located in either[26]

1. A rural Health Professional Shortage Area, either located outside of an MSA or in a rural census tract, as determined by the Office of Rural Health Policy within the HRSA; or
2. A county outside of an MSA.

Although interpreting these requirements has been a source of confusion in the past, HHS has developed a streamlined method for providers, including Tele-ICU providers, to determine if the location of the proposed facility receiving telehealth services meets this geographic requirement.[31,32] The Medicare Telehealth Payment Eligibility Analyzer is available at http://datawarehouse.hrsa.gov/telehealthAdvisor/telehealthEligibility.aspx.

Unfortunate for Tele-ICU providers is that this restriction, permitting reimbursement for only those telehealth services provided in rural areas, prohibits programs in urban areas from obtaining any reimbursement for Tele-ICU services from Medicare. This limitation exists regardless of whether or not other Medicare conditions for telehealth reimbursement are met.

In addition to this geographic restriction on telehealth reimbursement from Medicare, there is only a specific set of eligible telehealth services that will be reimbursed after all other conditions of payment are met. This list includes emergency and inpatient consultation services, follow-up inpatient and consultations, and subsequent hospital care services (with the limitation of 1 telehealth visit every 3 days), among other services. The list of eligible services, however, does not include critical care services. Because of this, Tele-ICU providers must determine the appropriate code for the service being provided based on the structure and design of the Tele-ICU program, and determine if the services being provided via telehealth meet the appropriate guidelines for billing Medicare.

Medicaid

According to the Center for Connected Health Policy's (CCHP) State Telehealth Laws and Reimbursement Policies report, "each state's laws, regulations, and Medicaid program policies differ significantly."[33] Of the 50 states and the District of Columbia that were examined by CCHP, it was found that 46 states have some form of reimbursement for telehealth in their program. Only Iowa, Massachusetts, New Hampshire, and Rhode Island lack any written policies related to telehealth reimbursement.

The 46 states that do provide reimbursement for telehealth services impact Tele-ICU reimbursement in different ways. In some cases, state Medicaid programs may provide comprehensive reimbursement for common Tele-ICU services, and in other cases, may not provide reimbursement for any common services. To determine what Tele-ICU services may be reimbursed by applicable state Medicaid programs, Tele-ICU providers can use the CCHP report as a guide to assist in accessing the then-current Medicaid reimbursement guidelines for telehealth services. Certain documents contained in the CCHP examination are more specific than others, but all can help illuminate the available Medicaid reimbursement for Tele-ICU providers in each state Medicaid program.

According to the ATA, there are a series of state Medicaid programs that have legislatively mandated Medicaid reimbursement for most services that are otherwise reimbursed in person.[34] These states presumably also fall into the 46 states the CCHP has reported as providing some form of reimbursement. These state Medicaid programs perhaps suggest a higher likelihood of available reimbursement for common Tele-ICU services due to this legal requirement to reimburse telehealth services.

Commercial: Private Insurance

Private insurance policies are regulated at the state level and therefore reimbursement guidelines can vary both by state and even by payer within that state.[35] There is also a growing trend of states that mandate private insurance companies to reimburse telehealth services if those same services are otherwise reimbursed when provided in person.[34] Even in states where no such mandates exist, there is growing evidence to suggest that private insurers in states have voluntarily adopted reimbursement policies for telehealth services.[35]

In states in which reimbursement is mandated, Tele-ICU providers should be able to submit claims with the appropriate services and telehealth modifiers to obtain payment for most services otherwise reimbursed in person. In states in which no such mandates exist, Tele-ICU providers should proactively review the policies, provider manuals, and fee schedules of the payers they commonly bill. Tele-ICU providers also should review contracts they have already executed with the payer, which may or may not reference the inclusion or exclusion of reimbursement for telehealth services.

Summary

Obtaining reimbursement for Tele-ICU services depends on geographic location, type of service, and clinical model. Combining the most widely available summarized information referenced in this article also may help identify states and regions that are most attractive to Tele-ICU reimbursement considering these sometimes competing factors and considerations (**Table 1**).

Steps for Success

Although there are often competing and/or contradicting telehealth reimbursement guidelines within each financial class, there are a few steps that Tele-ICU providers can take to simplify the process to help determine if billing should be pursued:

1. Document the most common services that are provided within the Tele-ICU program and document the most appropriate, nonpayer-specific billing code for that service.
2. Visit the Medicare Telehealth Payment Eligibility Analyzer is at http://datawarehouse. hrsa.gov/telehealthAdvisor/telehealthEligibility.aspx to determine if the proposed

Table 1
Telehealth reimbursement by state

State	Medicaid Reimbursement for Telehealth Services in Some Form (as of February 2014)[33]	Mandated Medicaid Reimbursement for Telehealth Services (as of July 30, 2014)[34]	Mandated Private Insurance Reimbursement for Telehealth Services (as of July 30, 2014)[34]
Alabama	Yes		
Alaska	Yes		Proposed
Arizona	Yes		Yes
Arkansas	Yes		
California	Yes	Yes	Yes
Colorado	Yes	Yes	Yes
Connecticut	Yes		Proposed
District of Columbia	Yes	Yes	Yes
Delaware	Yes		
Florida	Yes	Proposed	Proposed
Georgia	Yes		Yes
Hawaii	Yes		Yes
Idaho	Yes		
Illinois	Yes		Proposed
Indiana	Yes	Yes	
Iowa		Proposed	Proposed
Kansas	Yes		
Kentucky	Yes	Yes	Yes
Louisiana	Yes	Proposed	Yes
Maine	Yes		Yes
Maryland	Yes	Yes	Yes
Massachusetts		Proposed	Proposed
Michigan	Yes		Yes
Minnesota	Yes	Yes	
Mississippi	Yes	Yes	Yes
Missouri	Yes	Proposed	Yes
Montana	Yes		Yes
Nebraska	Yes	Yes	Proposed
Nevada	Yes		
New Hampshire			Yes
New Jersey	Yes		
New Mexico	Yes		Yes
New York	Yes	Proposed	Proposed
North Carolina	Yes		
North Dakota	Yes		
Ohio	Yes	Yes	Proposed
Oklahoma	Yes	Proposed	Yes
Oregon	Yes		Yes
Pennsylvania	Yes		Proposed

(continued on next page)

Table 1 *(continued)*			
State	Medicaid Reimbursement for Telehealth Services in Some Form (as of February 2014)[33]	Mandated Medicaid Reimbursement for Telehealth Services (as of July 30, 2014)[34]	Mandated Private Insurance Reimbursement for Telehealth Services (as of July 30, 2014)[34]
Rhode Island		Proposed	Proposed
South Carolina	Yes		Proposed
South Dakota	Yes		
Tennessee	Yes	Yes	Yes
Texas	Yes	Yes	Yes
Utah	Yes		
Vermont	Yes	Yes	Yes
Virginia	Yes		Yes
Washington	Yes	Proposed	Proposed
West Virginia	Yes	Proposed	Proposed
Wisconsin	Yes		
Wyoming	Yes		

facility location(s) for the Tele-ICU program meet the rural requirement for Medicare reimbursement.

3. Reference the Medicare Learning Network document summarizing Medicare telehealth reimbursement guidelines to determine if the Tele-ICU program, including the billing codes most commonly provided within the program, meet the requirements for Medicare reimbursement.

4. Use the CCHP report referenced in this article as a guide to assist in accessing the then-current Medicaid reimbursement guidelines for telehealth services in the appropriate states. Determine if the Tele-ICU program, including the billing codes most commonly provided within the program, meet the requirements for Medicaid reimbursement.

5. Reference the ATA's state legislation tracker to determine if the Tele-ICU program is located in a state that mandates reimbursement from private insurance. If the state does not mandate reimbursement, contact each high-volume payer to determine reimbursement guidelines for telehealth services.

6. Consider researching and/or obtaining fee schedules for all of the major payers that indicate available reimbursement for telehealth services to determine the expected fee schedule payment amount for each telehealth service provided in the Tele-ICU program.

7. When Tele-ICU program patient volume is known, including the percentage of patient volume in each major financial class, estimate expected Tele-ICU reimbursement by payer by combining fee schedule amounts with expected program volume for each financial class. Add the expected reimbursement amounts for each payer to determine total program reimbursement.

REFERENCES

1. Reynolds N, Rogove H, Bander J, et al. A working lexicon for the tele-intensive care unit: we need to define tele-intensive care unit to grow and understand it. Telemed J E Health 2011;17(10):773–83.

2. Rogove HJ, McArthur D, Demaerschalk BM, et al. Barriers to telemedicine: survey of current users in acute care units. Telemed J E Health 2012;18(1):48–53.

3. Lipson R, Henderson TM. State initiatives to promote telemedicine. Telemed J 1996;2(2):109–22.

4. Jacobson PD, Selvin E. Licensing telemedicine: the need for a national system. Telemed J E Health 2000;6(4):429–40.

5. Office for the Advancement of Telehealth. Telemedicine Licensure Report. 2003. Available at: http://www.hrsa.gov/ruralhealth/about/telehealth/licenserpt03.pdf. Accessed July 15, 2014.

6. Wakefield MK. HRSA Health Licensing Board Report to Congress. Senate Report 111–166. Available at: http://www.hrsa.gov/ruralhealth/about/telehealth/licenserpt10.pdf. Accessed May 26, 2014.

7. Nursing State Licensure Compact. Available at: http://nursingworld.org/MainMenuCategories/Policy-Advocacy/State/Legislative-Agenda-Reports/Licensure Compact. Accessed May 26, 2014.

8. Cwiek MA, Rafiq A, Qamar A, et al. Policy telemedicine licensure in the United States: the need for a cooperative regional approach. Telemed J E Health 2007;13(2):141–7.

9. Ferrer DC, Yellowlees PM. Telepsychiatry: licensing and professional boundary concerns. Virtual Mentor 2012;14(6):477–82.

10. Telehealth Improvement Act of 2004. Available at: https://beta.congress.gov/bill/108th-congress/senate-bill/2325. Accessed July 5, 2014.

11. STEP ACT 2011: H.R. 1832 (112th): Servicemembers' Telemedicine and E-Health Portability Act of 2011. Available at: http://www.govtrack.us/congress/bills/112/hr1832/text. Accessed July 14. 2014.

12. Veterans E-Health & Telemedicine Support Act of 2013: H.R. 2001. Available at: https://www.govtrack.us/congress/bills/113/hr2001. Accessed July 5, 2014.

13. TELE-MED Act of 2013: H.R. 3077. Available at: https://beta.congress.gov/bill/113th-congress/house-bill/3077. Accessed July 5, 2014.

14. Telehealth Enhancement Act of 2013: H.R. 3306. Available at: https://beta.congress.gov/bill/113th-congress/house-bill/3306. Accessed July 5, 2014.

15. Telehealth Modernization of 2013: H.R. 3750. Available at: https://www.govtrack.us/congress/bills/113/hr3750/text. Accessed July 5, 2014.

16. Medicare Telehealth Parity Act of 2014: H.R. 5380. Available at: https://www.govtrack.us/congress/bills/113/hr5380?utm_campaign=govtrack_feed&utm_source=govtrack/feed&utm_medium=rss. Accessed August 6, 2014.

17. Telehealth Enhancement Act 2014: S. 2662. Available at: https://www.govtrack.us/congress/bills/113/s2662. Accessed August 6, 2014.

18. Bashur R. Telemedicine and state-based licensure in the United States, revisited. Telemed J E Health 2008;14(4):310–1.

19. ATA Medical licensure and practice requirements, 2011. Available at: http://www.americantelemed.org/docs/default-source/policy/ata-policy-on-state-medical-licensure-and-practice-requirements.pdf?sfvrsn=10. Accessed August 16, 2014.

20. American Bar Association Health Law Section Report to the House of Delegate 2008. Available at: http://www.americanbar.org/content/dam/aba/migrated/health/04_government_sub/media/116B_Tele_Final.authcheckdam.pdf. Accessed July 5, 2014.

21. ATA FixLicensure. Available at: http://www.americantelemed.org/fixlicensure-org#.U0VEDF7Nwlo. Accessed July 5, 2014.

22. Available at: https://www.fsmb.org/Media/Default/PDF/Advocacy/Compact%20Draft%20Language%20July%202014.pdf. Accessed August 1, 2014.

23. Billings, Greg T. "Credentialing and Privileging: Proposed Rule from the Centers for Medicare and Medicaid Service." Center for Telehealth and e-Health Law 1.1 (2010). Available at: http://telehealthpolicy.us/credentialing-privileging. Accessed July 20, 2014.

24. CMS ruling on telemedicine credentialing, 2011. Available at: http://telehealthpolicy.us/credentialing-privileging. Accessed July 1, 2014.

25. Payne S L, Everett W. Planning for Tele-ICU in California. Report to the California Healthcare Foundation 2011. Available at: www.intouchhealth.com/2011%20NEHI-Tele%20ICU%20Report.pdf. Accessed July 22, 2014.

26. Department of Health and Human Services: Rural Health Fact Sheet Series: Telehealth Services. Available at: http://www.cms.gov/Outreach-and-Education/Medicare-Learning-Network-MLN/MLNProducts/downloads/telehealthsrvcsfctsht.pdf. Accessed August 8, 2014.

27. Medicare Physician Fee Schedule - overview. https://www.cms.gov/apps/physician-fee-schedule/overview.aspx. Accessed August 8, 2014.

28. Medicaid.gov: Telemedicine. Available at: http://www.medicaid.gov/Medicaid-CHIP-Program-Information/By-Topics/Delivery-Systems/Telemedicine.html Accessed August 8, 2014.

29. CTel Robert J Waters Center for Telehealth & e-Health Law: Medicaid reimbursement. http://ctel.org/expertise/reimbursement/medicaid-reimbursement/. Accessed August 8, 2014.

30. CTel Robert J Waters Center for Telehealth & e-Health Law: Reimbursement overview. http://ctel.org/expertise/reimbursement/reimbursement-overview/. Accessed August 8, 2014.

31. CTel Robert J Waters Center for Telehealth & e-Health Law: How to determine if your telehealth originating site is rural? http://ctel.org/2013/01/how-to-determine-if-your-telehealth-originating-site-is-rural/#. Accessed August 8, 2014.

32. Medicare Telehealth Payment Eligibility Analyzer. Available at: http://datawarehouse.hrsa.gov/telehealthAdvisor/telehealthEligibility.aspx. Accessed August 8, 2014.

33. Center for Connected Health Policy: State Telehealth Laws and Reimbursement Policies February 2014. Available at: http://telehealthpolicy.us/sites/telehealthpolicy.us/files/uploader/50-State%20February%202014%20-%20Correct%20Grant%20Numbers.pdf. Accessed August 8, 2014.

34. American Telemedicine Association 2014 State Telemedicine Legislation Tracking. Available at: http://www.americantelemed.org/docs/default-source/policy/state-telemedicine-policy-matrix.pdf?sfvrsn=44. Accessed August 8, 2014.

35. Antoniotti N, Drude K, Rowe N. Private payer telehealth reimbursement in the United States. Telemed J E Health 2014;20(6):539–43.

Options for Tele-Intensive Care Unit Design: Centralized Versus Decentralized and Other Considerations

It Is Not Just a "Another Black Sedan"

H. Neal Reynolds, MD[a],*, Joseph J. Bander, MD[b]

KEYWORDS

- Tele-ICU • Design • Technology • ICU

KEY POINTS

- The decision to acquire and develop Tele-ICU technology should be thoughtful, educated, and consider many of the variables presented.
- Belief in predicted return on investment may falter with time and lead to withdrawal of administrative support, particularly with more expensive programs.
- Failure to develop the medical workforce in a sustainable fashion could lead to failure or additional expenses when hiring intermediary programs.
- If a restrictive Tele-ICU technology is adopted, future growth plans could be stunted and the full value of the technology not realized.

INTRODUCTION

Henry Ford built his first "quadracycle" in 1896. It was another 27 years before the invention of the assembly line, in December 13, 1913, when Ford began to produce the Model T in large numbers.[1,2] The production time fell from more than 12 hours to 93 minutes. The innovation depended on using identical and interchangeable parts. Therefore, the first Model Ts were generally identical; there was no variation. The buyer

---

Financial Disclosure: H.N. Reynolds: No current financial disclosures. Previously a paid employee with VISICU in 2000–2001. Served on the advisory board for InTouch Health 2004–2008, completed grant funded research, 2010, and participated in the InTouch Health Research Consortium, all without financial remuneration.

[a] Division of Critical Care Medicine, R Adams Cowley Shock Trauma Center, University of Maryland Medical Center, University of Maryland School of Medicine, 22 South Greene Street, Baltimore, MD 21201, USA; [b] St Joseph Mercy Health System-Ann Arbor, 5301 McAuley Drive, Ypsilanti, MI 48197, USA
* Corresponding author.
E-mail address: HNeal.Reynolds@gmail.com

Crit Care Clin 31 (2015) 335–350
http://dx.doi.org/10.1016/j.ccc.2014.12.010
0749-0704/15/$ – see front matter © 2015 Elsevier Inc. All rights reserved.

was left with 1 option: a Model T or none at all. Now, in 2014, there are more than 44 new car brands available in the United States alone,[3] each with multiple models (Ford with 40 models) and each model with "comfort options," "entertainment options," "safety options," "appearance options," and "performance options."[4] The choice among all these brands, models, and options does not require technical expertise, such as engine compression ratio or gearing in the differential, just a definition of preferences and characteristics. Similarly, the Tele-ICU has evolved, although not nearly as dramatically as the automobile. Either way, there are significant choices to be made, beyond buying the generic early versions. This article is designed to consider some of those options.

HISTORY OF THE TELE-INTENSIVE CARE UNIT

Telemedicine was introduced into the intensive care unit (ICU) in the 1970s via early efforts of Grundy and colleagues.[5,6] Subsequently, telemedicine in the ICU has grown exponentially after the first commercial installation in Norfolk, Virginia, occurred in 2000.[7,8] The driving force for the expansion of telemedicine in the ICU evolved from a manpower maldistribution[9,10] shortage within the field of critical care,[11–15] growing value of intensivists,[16–19] recommendations from the Leapfrog group,[20] successes systematizing critical care and the telemedicine in the ICU,[7,8] and support for increasing telemedicine as part of Health Care reform.[21–23] Furthermore, data are emerging that the intensivist can have a significant positive impact on outcomes of critically ill patients when utilizing telemedicine technologies.[7,8,24,25] The literature evaluating Tele-ICU has evolved such that there are now 2 meta-analyses available,[26,27] both of which suggest lower ICU mortality after implementation of a Tele-ICU. Of note, Wilcox and Adhikari[27] conclude that the final structural model remains undefined. All of these data are supplemented by a recent, functional review of the literature[28]; it seems that the Tele-ICU is here to stay.

The Telemedicine examination is visual and not hands on, other than surrogate examinations from on-site nursing. Skeptics have suggested that the lack of a hands-on examination is a critical lack, but data are evolving that the visual examination and visual review of graphical waveforms improves accuracy of decision making.[29,30] There are multiple reports suggesting better compliance with evidence-based medical protocols when a centralized telemedicine process is in place.[31–37] Finally, although it seems intuitive, evidence has evolved that telemedicine in the ICU may have even greater impact in the rural environment.[38–41]

From 2000 to 2010, a single vendor and single design have largely driven growth. To stimulate alternative modalities and designs, a group of national experts in the field of Tele-ICU medicine published a "LEXICON" for the Tele-ICU.[42] The concept was simply to stimulate better descriptive language such that the new participants would ask for more specific design elements. This was followed by an examination of staffing processes[43] designed to expand the associated language and options for different staffing models.

To date, there have been no head-to-head evaluations of the various alternative technologies, networking models, or staffing structures for the Tele-ICU. It remains unclear what informational elements are mandatory to facilitate best diagnostic and therapeutic decisions in the Tele-ICU or what elements are unnecessary, superfluous, or just overengineered.

CONSIDERATIONS PRE-IMPLEMENTATION FOR THE TELE-INTENSIVE CARE UNIT

Before describing some specifics of the Tele-ICU, the following questions should be considered when initiating a Tele-ICU program. The authors have offered caveats suggesting potential outcomes and/or barriers. Thoroughly considering these questions preemptively may yield a successful program in the long term, versus one that encounters internal hospital political or economic turbulence and ultimately fails.

Assess Finances

- Today, and in a changing health care environment (hospital total patient revenue, global reimbursement, accountable care organizations, patient-centered medical homes), how will new reimbursement schemes impact hospital incentives?
- Stability of leadership should be assessed. Chief executive officers (CEOs) change their minds, change support, or change jobs, causing future support to change or completely erode.
- Will the return on investment (ROI) be sustainable and enough to support the program in the long term?
- Will the program be dependent on significant, fee-for-service reimbursement for survival?
- If reimbursement is important, the developer should assess local payers and payer mix (Medicare, Medicaid, and commercial payers) before completion of the financial model.

Caveats

1. Total patient revenue or global reimbursement schemes[44] have removed incentives to attract new patients to major hub hospitals and have dissuaded community total patient revenue hospitals from sending patients to more expensive hub hospitals. Therefore, total patient revenue may serve to dissuade an organization from adopting a Tele-ICU. It is important to know what payer model your facility is involved with, both currently and in the foreseeable future.
2. Accountable care organizations are effectively supported by the Centers for Medicare and Medicaid Services, capitated programs that disincentivize hospital admissions and may reduce future needs for ICU care.[45] The developer should be aware of the local penetration of the accountable care organizations reimbursement model.
3. The average "life expectancy" of a hospital CEO is about 5.5 years with 14% to 18%[46] yearly change over. So-called long-term decisions made by a current CEO may not carry through to subsequent CEOs. Seek support beyond the CEO.
4. Large, centralized programs depend on full funding from the parent facility with the expectation that the facility will benefit from ROI through cost savings.[40,47] Be sure that the institution believes in the projected ROI.
5. If independent financial sustainability is important, system designers should investigate local and national reimbursement.[48] Reimbursement through the Medicare system is much more limited[49-51] with only nonreimbursable, "class III–ICD" critical care billing codes.

Assess Human Resources: Medical Doctors

- Do you need medical doctors (MDs) or could critical care trained nurses or midlevel practitioners suffice?
- Will your current cadre of intensivists participate (or refuse to participate) in a new Tele-ICU program?
- Can you recruit (and retain) physicians to staff the Tele-ICU?
- Can a Tele-ICU program afford dedicated intensivists, nurses, or midlevel practitioners?
- How much do you want to involve the consulting MDs into the Tele-ICU?

Caveats

1. Eastern Maine Medical Center initially ran a Tele-ICU program without MD involvement and were able to demonstrate a positive impact on patient outcomes (personal communication from Mary McCarthy, Director, Tele-ICU program at Eastern Maine Medical Center, 2011).
2. The more rural the Tele-ICU, the more difficult to recruit and retain intensivists.[52] But even urban areas experience difficulty, with recruitment driving the growth of a middle-man industry that provides staffing to the Tele-ICU.[53]
3. Staffing with MDs, registered nurses (RNs), or midlevel professionals accounts for about 72% of ongoing operating costs.[54] Providing a single MD, 12 hours per day, 365 days per year at $200 per hour accrues a cost of $876,000 per year. As a consequence, some programs are investigating alternative staffing models.
4. Consulting physicians, such as nephrologists and cardiologists, are outside the telecommunications system when the Tele-ICU program utilizes a closed architecture system, but may access the real-time audio–video connection with the open architecture systems.[42] Preemptive decisions regarding utilization of community physicians and consultants will drive the decision to deploy the open versus the closed architecture system.

Assess Human Resources: Registered Nurses

- Will your current cadre of critical care nurses participate in the Tele-ICU?
- How will you maintain nursing bedside expertise?
- How can Tele-ICU nursing prestige be maintained to avoid relegation to a perceived second class stature?

Caveats

1. Evaluating nursing Tele-ICU competencies and establishing a thorough orientation is likely to overcome nursing anxiety of moving to a new and unknown working environment.[55]
2. The Tele-ICU nurse should initially have significant bedside experience before becoming a Tele-ICU nurse.[56] Some programs require an ongoing minimum of bedside nursing practice time.
3. The formal "CCRN-e" accreditation was established and serves to lend prestige and recognition to the field of Tele-ICU nursing and may serve to maintain stability in the workforce.[57,58] All Tele-ICU nurses should be encouraged to seek the CCRN-e certificate.

Define Goals of Program

- Will the Tele-ICU program provide coverage to internal ICUs within the parent facility only?
- Will the Tele-ICU program provide outreach to community ICUs?
- Is the intent of the Tele-ICU program to develop a network of ICUs with centripetal (community to the center hub) and/or centrifugal (from center hub toward community) movement of patients?
- To avoid future dissatisfaction, preemptively define Tele-ICU coverage: 24 hours a day versus 8 to 12 hours a day versus reactive consultative only.
- Will the Tele-ICU program provide coverage only when on-site intensivists are not present?

Caveats

1. When more complex and expensive technology is selected, it may be necessary to spread the cost across multiple ICUs. When considering less expensive or less complex technology, single unit coverage becomes financially feasible.
2. Many, if not all, programs are designed to provide service only when the "on-site" intensivist are off site and/or unavailable.
3. "Continuous" care is rarely continuous 24 × 7 but rather, continuous for limited numbers of hours per day such as 8 or 12 hours per day. Alternatively, certain aspects may be continuous, 24 × 7 such as nursing Tele-ICU monitoring; intensivist monitoring could be limited to 8 to 12 hours per day.
4. Tele-ICU technology can support both centripetal (typical patient flow from community to hub) and centrifugal (repatriation to the community). Repatriation to the community can facilitate more efficient utilization of the high-end hub ICU beds.

Technical Support and Guidelines

- Will the Tele-ICU vendor provide all technical support?
- Will the hospital Information Technology department participate in the installation and ongoing technical support?
- Does the Tele-ICU vendor provide real-time, 24 × 7, technical support?
- Certain vendors have scheduled mid-day, "down time" for maintenance and upgrades. The designer should understand the impact of "down time" on the flow of patient care and consider alternative documentation monitoring modalities

Caveats

1. Establishment of a Tele-ICU will always require considerable collaboration between the vendor and the local medical facility's Information Technology group. Defining clear lines of responsibility is mandatory before "going live," and preferably before installation. A point of contention is frequently the interface between the wireless system (or hospital backbone) and the Tele-ICU equipment.
2. The American Telemedicine Association has recently established Guidelines for Tele-ICU Operations with recommended minimums.[59] These guidelines are weighted toward certain technologies, but serve as a beginning reference.
3. Essentially, all major software requires periodic updates and upgrades. Some do so by temporarily ceasing functionality and without an alternative mechanism to continue to perform routine duties. This should be understood in advance with alternative care models put in place before going live.

Institutional Politics

- What are the driving forces for the development of a Tele-ICU program?
- Determine where resistance lies and what the origin of resistance is to the development of a Tele-ICU.

Caveats

1. Tele-ICU program development driven only by hospital administration for stated cost savings or quality purposes, without a buy-in from the physician staff, are doomed to serious turbulence if not failure. Bring all stakeholders to the table early.

2. Rotating clinicians from bedside work to remote Tele-ICU service increases exposure to both sides of the service model and may reduce the "us versus them" stigma.[60]
2. Exclusion of subspecialists from direct access to the Tele-ICU technology may increase resistance. Conversely, inclusion of the subspecialists to the technology may greatly improve local physician buy-in.

Quality Metrics

- What quality metrics do you currently monitor?[59]
- Do you need additional metrics?
- Should those metrics come from the Tele-ICU database or via current ICU sources?
- Will a Tele-ICU database and analysis cost more than using current data collection technologies?
- Will the Tele-ICU database and analysis be as good as or better than the current analysis?

Caveats

1. Quality metrics should at least include the traditional metrics, such as mortality, length of stay, ventilator duration of use, and infectious complications, but should also include quality metrics related to the unique performance of telemedicine, such as patient and family acceptance of telemedicine interventions, system scheduled and unscheduled downtime, quality of the audio and video, remote care provider response time, and remote care provider perceived competence.[59]
2. If a facility already has a staff of well-qualified data analysts and data collectors who provide a wide range of hospital quality metrics, there may be little savings in shifting quality analysis to a Tele-ICU service provided by an outside vendor.

What Future Growth Pattern for the Tele-Intensive Care Unit

- Does the program vision include vertical growth (vertical scaling) with continued expansion of the same service line?
- Does the program vision include horizontal growth (horizontal scaling) with expansion into other fields of service?[61]

Caveats

1. The centralized Tele-ICU is ideally suited for vertical growth with inclusion of more critical care programs by expansion of same line of services with more intensivist and critical care nursing staffing.
2. Horizontal scaling mandates an "open architecture"[42] as defined elsewhere in this article. Open architecture technology is necessary to support access by multiple specialists who will not be based in a centralized, closed architecture program (**Fig. 1**)

Regional Technical Limitations

- What are the current limitations on the local, wireless, or broadband service?
- What are the limitations on the local "hard-wired" broadband service?
- Could some of the rural facilities be subject to the expenses of "the last mile"?

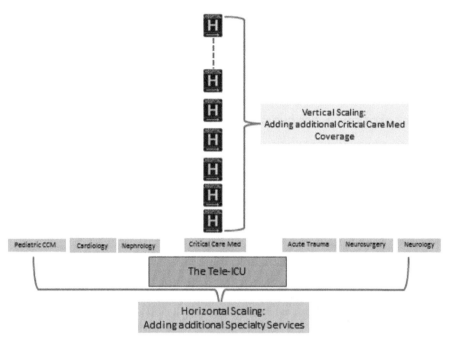

Fig. 1. Vertical scaling with addition of more critical care units for the provision of critical care support only. Horizontal scaling entails the addition of additional service lines such as suggested to include cardiology, trauma, and neurology.

Caveats

1. Certain technologies necessary to facilitate an "open architecture" capability will require significant wireless broad band capabilities, which may not be available regionally.[62] Such limitations could restrict the development of multispecialty based Tele-ICU.
2. Rural communities suffer from significant shortage of wired broadband technology. The problem is of such a magnitude as to have provoked the development of a government-based Broadband Initiative Program.[63]
3. Multiple state and federal initiatives have supported the development of high-speed "back-bone" networks to rural communities. The final connection from the back-bone to a consumer or facility is referred to as the "last mile" where "mile" is metaphorical for a relatively short distance. Costs to connect from a regional broadband backbone can be significant and should be understood and incorporated into any financial planning[64] and startup costs

Additional Technical Burdens on the Staff

- Does a Tele-ICU technology increase the burden of documentation (double documentation) for the critical care staff?
- If so, will double documentation require additional staff such as scribes?

Caveats

1. Certain Tele-ICU programs have ICU-focused Electronic Medical Record (EMR) systems deployed in the real ICU that may not interface with the hospital EMR.

Intensivist staff could be required to document in both systems, thereby increasing workload and resistance to adoption.
2. Despite vendor reports, some Tele-ICU EMR (at the real ICU) can be seen as burdensome. As a result, the ICU staff may request supplemental scribe staff to deal with the workload, as is done in emergency departments.[65]

TWO KEY DECISIONS IN DESIGNING A TELE-INTENSIVE CARE UNIT

Once having considered all these issues, a key question will be whether the Tele-ICU should be centralized or decentralized. Part and parcel to this question is the decision regarding communications systems based on an "open" versus a "closed" architecture. Centralized or decentralized Tele-ICUs have been defined elsewhere[42] and are reiterated herein. The definition is provided as a pure description knowing that, with evolution and time, some systems will have characteristics of both centralized and decentralized programs (hybrid programs).

The Centralized Tele-Intensive Care Unit

A centralized Tele-ICU is a hub-and-spoke model in which critical care services originate from a hub and services are delivered at a spoke facility. The hub (or center) is an established site with staffing that includes intensivists, nurses, and clerical and technical staff. The established hub is connected to 1 or multiple medical facilities and/or multiple ICUs. As such, the intensivists must work from the central hub and not from other sites. Therefore, the centralized Tele-ICU is a discrete site and has an established process of care.

The Decentralized Tele-Intensive Care Unit

In this model, there is no defined, established central monitoring facility or staff dedicated to being present at any remote site. The decentralized model typically involves computers or mobile devices equipped with camera, speakers, and microphones located at sites of convenience such as physician offices, homes, or mobile sites. Therefore, the decentralized Tele-ICU is not a specific or single site, but more of a process.

Open Architecture

A flexible, undedicated communications system that supports connectivity by 1 or more care providers, from 1 or more sites, to 1 or multiple sites. Open architecture generally implies connectivity via the Internet. Open architecture networks may take any of the following forms:

a. Single physician to a single site with multiple patients: One physician (from home, office, or mobile device) providing critical care services to 1 ICU and providing care for any or all the patients within that ICU.
b. Single physician to multiple sites and/or multiple patients: An individual physician could be virtually present, sequentially, at several different medical sites from a home, office, or mobile device and provide services for some or all patients at each site.
c. Multiple physicians from multiple sites to a single patient: Multiple physicians could simultaneously evaluate a single patient, each physician located at a separate location.
d. Multiple physicians from multiple sites to multiple sites and multiple patients.

Closed Architecture

A closed architecture Tele-ICU program has point-to-point, dedicated communication to a patient from a central monitoring facility. For purity of definition, there would be no option for physicians outside the closed system to have full access to patient audio–video, clinical, or trending information. Medical consultants would be functionally external to the closed Tele-ICU system and could only evaluate a patient via traditional communications, such as the telephone. The closed architecture model generally employs dedicated high-speed lines. Functionally, the closed architecture exists outside the Internet, although internal data may be transmitted over high-speed cables or fibers by using internet protocol.

In discussing generalities about technology, the intent is to remain vendor neutral. The centralized Tele-ICUs may be based on the Philips VISICU technology (Andover, MA, USA), Cerner EMR/Technology (Kansas City, MO, USA), IMDSoft (Dedham, MA, USA), or EPIC (Verona, WI, USA). Conversely, decentralized Tele-ICUs may be based on the Intouch Health robotic (Santa Barbara, CA, USA) technology, or any of the web-based carts to include Polycom (San Jose, CA, USA), AMD Global (Chelmsford, MA, USA), and Rubbermaid (Huntersville, NC, USA). However, the vast majority of the centralized Tele-ICUs deploy the Philips VISICU system (positioned in approximately 400 hospitals nationwide) and the vast majority of the decentralized Tele-ICU systems are based on the InTouch Health web-enabled, wireless robotic technology (positioned in about 950 hospitals in North America).

THE TELE-INTENSIVE CARE UNIT LITERATURE: CENTRALIZED VERSUS DECENTRALIZED

To further define characteristics of systems, we have defined characteristics of the literature. A literature search was performed using the National Institutes of Health PubMed service and Google Scholar, using key words of Telemedicine, ICU, tele-ICU, Robots and Tele-ICU, ICU and Telemedicine with the intent to generally examine the literature for characteristics that define centralized versus decentralized Tele-ICUs. In general, if an article described the use of mobile devices that were stated or known to be web enabled, then the system was assumed to be decentralized with an open architecture communications system. If an article refers to a telemedicine center, a system hub, a "hub-and-spoke" functionality, or uses the phrase "telemedicine center," then the article was judged to refer to a centralized program. No assumptions were made about the connectivity (open vs closed architecture) unless specifically stated.

Overall, there is much more current literature describing centralized programs than decentralized programs in a ratio of about 3:1 (34 vs 12). Eight review articles were discovered that also generally focused on centralized programs. Ten articles were categorized as administrative in that the content was directed at establishing function, training, and nursing competencies, but again the majority of the focus was on centralized programs (**Table 1**). Based on a review of the relevant literature, combined with knowledge of the technology and clinical field, **Table 2** was created to help the reader understand the spectrum of differences between centralized versus decentralized tele-ICU technology (see **Table 2**).

Table 1			
Categorization of literature search related to the Tele-ICU			
Centralized Tele-ICU Publication	**Decentralized Tele-ICU Publication**	**Tele-ICU Administrative Related**	**Tele-ICU Review or Meta-Analysis**
Refs.[5,6,8,24,25,31–40,66–84]	Refs.[7,29,30,85–93]	Refs.[42,43,51–53,55–58,94,95]	Refs.[22,26–28,47,54,60,96,97]

Table 2
General comparison of the decentralized versus the centralized models for the Tele-ICU

Characteristic	Centralized Tele-ICU	Decentralized Tele-ICU
Open Architecture	Possible	Mandatory
Closed architecture	Most common model	Not workable
Requires dedicated communication lines (T-1, T-3, etc)	Yes: vendor dependent	No: Internet enabled
Real physical Tele-ICU site	Yes	Maybe/no
Vertical scaling	Good model for vertical scaling	Poor model for vertical scaling
Horizontal scaling	Poor model for horizontal scaling unless involves open architecture connectivity to specialists	Good model for horizontal scaling with open architecture
Cost of install	Higher	Lower
Operational costs	Higher	Lower
Complexity of install	Higher	Lower
Data gathering/analysis	Robust	Undefined
Smart alarms	Yes: vendor dependent	No: Bedside nurse functions as the "smart alarm"
Concurrent EMR	Generally yes, vendor dependent	Generally no: use local, preexisting EMR
MD provider mobility	None unless system incorporates open architecture	Greater mobility
MD provider flexibility	None: Care provider must be situated in the Tele-ICU	Greater flexibility, care provider can be mobile
RN provider mobility	None	N/A: Generally does not require dedicated RNs
RN provider flexibility	None	N/A: Generally does not require dedicated RNs
Provides "continuous" care	Yes: model dependent may be 24 h × 7, 12 h × 7 or 8 h × 7	No; rare exceptions
Provides "reactive" or "consultative" care	Yes	Yes
Provides "scheduled" care	Yes	Yes
Impact on other hospital ICU personnel	High	Low

Abbreviations: EMR, electronic medical record; MD, medical doctor; RN, registered nurse; T-1, dedicated telecommunications line, bandwidth 1.544 mb/s, cost = $1,000–$3,000/month; T-3, dedicated telecommunications line, bandwidth 43.233 mb/s, Cost ≥$3,000/mth.[98]

SUMMARY

The decision to acquire and develop Tele-ICU technology should be thoughtful, educated, and consider many of the variables discussed herein. Belief in predicted ROI may falter with time and lead to withdrawal of administrative support, particularly with more expensive programs. Failure to develop the medical workforce in a sustainable fashion could lead to failure or additional expenses when hiring intermediary programs. If a restrictive Tele-ICU technology is adopted, future growth plans could be stunted and the full value of the technology not realized. Finally, it is extraordinarily difficult to predict the evolution of the health care system and therefore to predict future reimbursement schemes.

Regarding the scientific literature, there are more comparative studies emanating from centralized programs although essentially all the studies are before versus after Tele-ICU implementation, unrandomized, and with large potential for confounding variables. Similar statements apply to studies/reports regarding decentralized programs. However, no study to date examines efficacy or cost effectiveness of centralized versus decentralized structured programs. By summary comparison, the centralized models offer:

- A turn-key, relatively full-service program;
- An EMR at the Tele-ICU end and the ICU end;
- Audio–video hardware and software;
- Mechanisms to accumulate and analyze data easily; and
- Virtual attendance at the bedside by intensivists assisted by virtual nursing presence.

The decentralized programs offer:

- The equivalent of placing the intensivist at the bedside;
- No need for all the associated support systems;
- Continued use of the hospital EMR and computerized physician order entry; and
- A reliance on established hospital programs to gather quality indicators and process the data.

The concept of centralized versus decentralized implies purity of definition. Unquestionably, hybrid models exist or will evolve, perhaps involving an established site ("bunker") with open architecture allowing outside physicians access to the telemedicine technology from virtually anywhere. As important is the concept of open versus closed architecture. Open architecture equates to "accessible" by multiple care providers, from multiple sites and can be done so with more than 1 remote care provider simultaneously. Closed architecture equates to restricted access limited only to those in the central site.

REFERENCES

1. Henry Ford Introduction of the Assembly line. Available at: http://history1900s.about.com/od/1910s/a/Ford–Assembly-Line.htm. Accessed July 8, 2014.
2. Ford's Assembly line starts rolling. Available at: http://history1900s.about.com/od/1910s/a/Ford–Assembly-Line.htm. Accessed July 8, 2014.
3. New cars. Available at: http://www.edmunds.com/new-cars. Accessed July 8, 2014.
4. Car options. Available at: http://www.cars.com/go/advice/. Accessed July 8, 2014.
5. Grundy BL, Jones PK, Lovitt A. Telemedicine in critical care: problems in design, implementation, and assessment. Crit Care Med 1982;10(7):471–5.
6. Grundy BL, Crawford P, Jones PK, et al. Telemedicine in critical care: an experiment in health care delivery. JACEP 1977;6(10):439–44.
7. Rosenfeld BA, Dorman T, Breslow MJ, et al. Intensive care unit telemedicine: alternate paradigm for providing continuous intensivist care. Crit Care Med 2000;28:3925–31.

8. Breslow MJ, Rosenfeld BA, Doerfler M, et al. Effect of a multiple-site intensive care unit telemedicine program on clinical and economic outcomes: an alternative paradigm for intensivist staffing. Crit Care Med 2004;32:31–8.
9. Kirch DG. How to fix the doctor shortage. Wall Street Journal 2010.
10. National Rural Health Association. Health care workforce distribution and shortage issues in rural America. Washington, DC: National Rural Health Association; 2003.
11. Angus DC, Kelley MA, Schmitz RJ, et al. Current and projected workforce requirements for care of the critical ill and patients with pulmonary disease: can we meet the requirements of an aging population? JAMA 2000;284:2762–70.
12. Health Resources and Services Administration Report to Congress. The critical care workforce: a study of the supply and demand for critical care physicians. Requested by: Senate Report 108–181. Available at: http://bhpr.hrsa.gov/healthworkforce/supplydemand/medicine/criticalcaresupply.pdf. Accessed January 12, 2015.
13. Kelley MA, Angus DC, Chalfin DB, et al. The critical care crisis in the United States: a report from the profession. Crit Care Med 2004;32:1219–22.
14. Grover A. Critical care workforce: a policy perspective. Crit Care Med 2006; 34(Suppl.3):S7–11.
15. Krell K. Critical care workforce. Crit Care Med 2008;36:1350–3.
16. Reynolds HN, Haupt MT, Carlson R. Impact of critical care physician staffing on patients with septic shock in a university medical care unit. JAMA 1988;260(33): 3446–50.
17. Li TC, Phillips MC, Shaw L, et al. On site physician staffing in a community hospital intensive care unit: impact on test and procedure use and on patient outcome. JAMA 1984;252:2023–7.
18. Young M, Birkmeyer J. Potential reduction in mortality rates using an intensivist model to manage intensive care units. Eff Clin Pract 2000;3:284–9.
19. Engoren M. The effect of prompt physician visits on intensive care unit mortality and cost. Crit Care Med 2005;33:727–32.
20. Leapfrog. Four leaps in hospital quality, safety and affordability. Available at: http://www.leapfroggroup.org. Accessed August 25, 2014.
21. Bashshur RL, Shannon GW, Krupinski EA, et al. National Telemedicine Initiatives: essential to Healthcare Reform. Telemedicine and e-Health 2009;15(6): 600–10.
22. New England Healthcare Institute, Massachusetts Technology Collaborative, Health Technology Center. Tele-ICUs: remote management in intensive care units. Cambridge (MA): New England Healthcare Institute; 2007.
23. Expansion of Medicare covered telemedicine services. p. 139–50. Available at: http://www.ofr.gov/OFRUpload/OFRData/2014-15948_PI.pdf. Accessed July 8, 2014.
24. Kohl B, Gutsche J, Kim P, et al. Effect of telemedicine on mortality and length of stay in a university ICU. Crit Care Med 2007;35(12):A22.
25. Shaffer JP, Breslow MJ, Johnson JW, et al. Remote ICU management improves outcomes in patients with cardio-pulmonary arrest. Crit Care Med 2005;33(12):A5.
26. Young LB, Chan PS, Lu X, et al. Impact of telemedicine intensive care unit coverage on patient outcomes: a systematic review and meta-analysis. Arch Intern Med 2011;171(6):498–506.
27. Wilcox ME, Adhikari NK. The effect of telemedicine in critically ill patients: systematic review and meta-analysis. Crit Care 2012;16(4):R127.
28. Deslich S, Coustasse A. Expanding technology in the ICU: the case for the utilization of telemedicine. Telemed J E Health 2014;20(5):1–8.

29. Vespa PM, Miller C, Hu X, et al. Intensive care unit robotic telepresence facilitates rapid physician response to unstable patients and decreased costs in a neurointensive care. Surg Neurol 2007;67:331–7.

30. Meyer BC, Ramen R, Hemmen T, et al. Efficacy of site-independent telemedicine in the STRokE DOC trial: a randomized, blinded, prospective study. Lancet Neuro 2008;7(9):787–95.

31. Youn BA. Utilizing robots and an ICU telemedicine program to provide intensivist support for rapid response teams. Chest 2006;130(4_Meeting abstracts):102s.

32. Patel B, Kao L, Thomas E, et al. Improving compliance with surviving sepsis campaign guidelines via remote electronic ICU monitoring. Crit Care Med 2007;35:A275.

33. Giessel GM, Leedom B. Centralized, remote ICU intervention improves best practices compliance. Chest 2007;132:444a.

34. Youn BA. ICU process improvement: using telemedicine to enhance compliance and documentation for the ventilator bundle. Chest 2006;130:226S.

35. Badawi O, Shemmeri E. Greater collaboration between remote intensivists and onsite clinicians improves best practice compliance. Crit Care Med 2006;34(12):A20.

36. Rincon T, Bourke G, Ikeda D. Centralized, remote care improves sepsis identification, bundle compliance and outcomes. Chest 2007;132:557S–8S.

37. Aaronson M, Zawada ET, Herr P. Role of a telemedicine intensive care unit program (TISP) on glycemic control (GC) in seriously ill patients in a rural health system. Chest 2006;130(Suppl):226S.

38. Zawada ET, Kapasla D, Herr P, et al. Prognostic outcomes after the initiation of an electronic telemedicine intensive care unit in a rural health system. S D Med 2006; 59:391–3.

39. Zawada E, Aaronson ML, Herr P, et al. Relationship between levels of consultative management and outcomes in a telemedicine intensivist staffing program (TISP) in a rural health system. Chest 2006;130:226S.

40. Zawada E, Herr P, Erickson D, et al. Financial benefit of a teleintensivist program to a rural health system. Chest 2007;132(4):444.

41. Burgiss SG. Telehealth technical assistance manual. Washington, DC: National Rural Health Association; 2006.

42. Reynolds HN, Rogove H, Bander J, et al. A working lexicon for the Tele-ICU: we need to define Tele-ICU to grow & understand it. Telemed J E Health 2011;17(10):773–83.

43. Reynolds HN, Bander J, McCarthy M. Different systems and formats for tele-ICU coverage. designing a tele-icu system to optimize functionality and investment. Crit Care Nurs Q 2012;35(4):1–14.

44. The Maryland Cost Services Review Commission. Maryland state total patient revenue reimbursement. Available at: http://www.hscrc.state.md.us/init_tpr.cfm. Accessed July 14, 2014.

45. Accountable care organizations. Available at: http://www.cms.gov/Medicare/Medicare-Fee-for-Service-Payment/ACO/. Accessed July 14, 2014.

46. American College of Healthcare Executives. Average tenure of hospital chief executive officers. Available at: https://www.ache.org/pubs/research/pdf/hospital_ceo_turnover_06.pdf. Accessed July 14, 2014.

47. Tele-ICU positive return on investment. Becky Rufo health affairs: at the intersection of health, healthcare and policy. Available at: http://content.healthaffairs.org/content/28/6/1859.2.full. Accessed July 14, 2014.

48. American Telemedicine Association. State Legislative Matrix. Available at: http://www.americantelemed.org/docs/default-source/policy/state-telemedicine-policy-matrix.pdf?sfvrsn=14. Accessed July 14, 2014.

49. Centers for Medicare and Medicaid Services (CMS). Telemedicine reimbursement. Available at: http://www.cms.gov/Outreach-and-Education/Medicare-Learning-Network-MLN/MLNProducts/downloads/telehealthsrvcsfctsht.pdf. Accessed July 14, 2014.

50. American Telemedicine Association. CMS reimbursement. Available at: http://www.americantelemed.org/docs/default-source/policy/medicare-payment-of-telemedicine-and-telehealth-services.pdf. Accessed July 14, 2014.

51. Reynolds HN. "Remote critical care services" in coding and billing. In: Dorman T, Britton F, Brown D, et al, editors. 6th edition. Society of Critical Care Medicine; 2014. p. 49–61.

52. Recruiting intensivists for the Veterans Administrations ICU. Available at: http://www.ruralhealth.va.gov/docs/issue-briefs/Tele-ICU-Implementation-032012.pdf. Accessed July 14, 2014.

53. Gorman MJ. Tele-ICU comes of age. Issues of recruiting intensivists to the Tele-ICU in health management technology. Available at: http://www.healthmgttech.com/articles/201112/tele-icu-comes-of-age.php. Accessed July 14, 2014.

54. Fifer S, Everett W, Adams M, et al. The Tele-ICU advisory Group and the FAST Tele-ICU Expert Panel. Critical Care, Critical Choices: the case for Tele-ICUs in Intensive Care. NEHI and Mass Technology Collaborative. Massachusetts, December, 2010. Available at: http://www.masstech.org/sites/mtc/files/documents/2010%20TeleICU%20Report.pdf. Accessed July 14, 2014.

55. Gorman MJ. A new view: tele–intensive care unit competencies. Available at: http://www.aacn.org/wd/Cetests/media/C115.pdf. Accessed July 14, 2014.

56. American Association of Critical-care Nurses. Tele-ICU Nursing practice guidelines. Available at: http://www.aacn.org/wd/practice/docs/tele-icu-guidelines.pdf. Accessed July 14, 2014.

57. American Association of Critical-care Nurses. CCRN-e certification: introduction. Available at: http://www.aacn.org/wd/certifications/content/ccrn-eintro.pcms?menu=certification. Accessed July 14, 2014.

58. Davis TM, Barden C, Olff C, et al. Professional accountability in the tele-ICU: the CCRN-E. Crit Care Nurs Q 2012;35(4):353–6.

59. American Telemedicine Association (ATA). ATA guidelines for Tele-ICU operations. 2014. Available at: http://www.americantelemed.org/docs/default-source/standards/guidelines-for-teleicu-operations.pdf?sfvrsn=2. Accessed July 14, 2014.

60. National Health Policy Institute (NEHI). NEHI Report: Tele-ICU poised for major growth in health care informatics. 2013. Available at: http://www.healthcare-informatics.com/news-item/nehi-report-tele-icu-poised-major-growth. Accessed July 14, 2014.

61. DNS Made Easy. Definition of vertical versus horizontal scaling. Available at: http://www.dnsmadeeasy.com/blog/vertical-and-horizontal-scaling/. Accessed July 14, 2014.

62. Strover S. Lack of broadband has crippling effect. 2011. Available at: http://www.utexas.edu/know/2011/04/08/strover_sharon_yonder/. Accessed July 14, 2014.

63. United States Department of Agriculture. Rural Utilities Service. Status of broadband initiatives program. Available at: http://www.rurdev.usda.gov/Reports/utp_RUS_BroadbandInitiativesProgram_Status_%20ReportApril2013.pdf. Accessed July 14, 2014.

64. Last Mile Technology. Available at: http://searchnetworking.techtarget.com/definition/last-mile-technology. Accessed July 14, 2014.

65. Medpage today. My experience with a scribe in the emergency department. Available at: http://www.kevinmd.com/blog/2012/12/experience-scribe-emergency-department.html. Accessed July 14, 2014.

66. Lilly CM, Cody S, Zhao H, et al. Hospital mortality, length of stay, and preventable complications among critically ill patients before and after tele-ICU reengineering of critical care processes. JAMA 2011;301(21):2175–83.

67. McCambridge M, Jones K, Paxton H, et al. Association of health information technology and teleintensivist coverage with decreased mortality and ventilator use in critically ill patients. Arch Intern Med 2010;170(7):648–53.

68. Morrison JL, Cai Q, Davis N, et al. Clinical and economic outcomes of the electronic intensive care unit: results from two community hospitals. Crit Care Med 2010;38(1):2–8.

69. Thomas EJ, Lucke JF, Wueste L, et al. Association of telemedicine for remote monitoring of intensive care patients with mortality, complications, and length of stay. JAMA 2009;302(24):2671–8.

70. Willmitch B, Golembeski S, Kim SS, et al. Clinical outcomes after telemedicine intensive care unit implementation. Crit Care Med 2012;40(2):450–4.

71. Lilly CM, McLaughlin JM, Zhao H, et al, for the UMass Memorial Critical Care Operations Group. A multi-center study of ICU telemedicine reengineering of adult critical care. Chest 2014;145(3):500–7. Available at: http://journal.publications.chestnet.org.

72. Lilly CM, Thomas EJ. Tele-ICU: experience to date. J Intensive Care Med 2010; 25:16–22.

73. Leong JR, Sirio CA, Rotondi AJ. eICU program favorably affect clinical and economic outcomes. Crit Care 2005;9(5):15–27.

74. Groves RH, Holcomb BW, Smith ML. Intensive care telemedicine: evaluating a model for proactive remote monitoring and intervention in the critical care setting. In: Latifi R, editor. Current principles and practices of telemedicine and e-health. Amsterdam: IOS Press; 2008. p. 131–46.

75. Chu-Weininger MY, Wueste L, Lucke JF, et al. The impact of a tele-ICU on provider attitudes about teamwork and safety climate. Qual Saf Health Care 2010;19:e39.

76. Khunlertkit A, Carayon P. Contributions of tele-intensive care unit (Tele-ICU) technology to quality of care and patient safety. J Crit Care 2013;28: 315.e1–12.

77. Franzini L, Sail KR, Thomas EJ, et al. Costs and cost-effectiveness of a telemedicine intensive care unit program in 6 intensive care units in a large health care system. J Crit Care 2011;26:329–34.

78. Wood D. Tele-ICU saves money as well as lives. Telemed J E Health 2011;17: 64–7.

79. Howell GH, Lem VM, Ball JM. Remote ICU care correlates with reduced health system mortality and length of stay outcomes. Chest 2007;132:138–45.

80. Rincon TA. Integration of evidence-based knowledge management in microsystems: a tele-ICU experience. Crit Care Nurs Q 2012;35:335–40.

81. Nassar BS, Vaughan-Sarrazin MS, Jiang L, et al. Impact of an intensive care unit telemedicine program on patient outcomes in an integrated health care system. JAMA Intern Med 2014;174(7):1160–7. http://dx.doi.org/10.1001/jamainternmed.2014.1503.

82. Fortis S, Weinert C, Bushinski R, et al. A tele-ICU program developed by academic intensivists: implementation, structure and cost details. Crit Care Med 2013;41(12) [abstract: 605].

83. Kruklitis RJ, Tracy JA, McCambridge MM. Clinical and financial considerations for implementing an ICU telemedicine program. Chest 2014;145(6):1392–6. http://dx.doi.org/10.1378/chest.13-0868.

84. Kumar S, Merchant S, Reynolds R. Tele-ICU: efficacy and cost-effectiveness approach of remotely managing the critical care. Open Med Inform J 2013;7: 24–9. Available at: http://www.ncbi.nlm.nih.gov/pmc/articles/PMC3785036/. Accessed July 15, 2014.

85. Reynolds EM, Grujovski A, Wright T, et al. Utilization of robotic "remote presence" technology within North American Intensive Care Units (ICUs). Telemed J E Health 2012;18(7):1–9.

86. Reynolds HN, Sheinfeld G, Chang J, et al. The Tele-ICU during a "disaster": seamless transition from routine operations to disaster mode. Telemed J E Health 2011;17(9):746–9.

87. Garingo A, Friedlich P, Tesoriero L, et al. The use of mobile robotic telemedicine technology in the neonatal intensive care unit. J Perinatol 2012;32(1):55–63.

88. Sapirstein A, Lone N, Latif A, et al. Tele ICU: paradox or panacea? Best Pract Res Clin Anaesthesiol 2009;23:115–26.

89. Sucher J, Todd SR, Jones SL, et al. Robotic telepresence: a helpful adjunct that is viewed favorably by critically ill surgical patients. Am J Surg 2011;202(6):843–7.

90. Rincon F, Vibbert M, Childs V, et al. Implementation of a model of robotic telepresence (RTP) in the neuro-ICU: effect on critical care nursing team satisfaction. NeuroCrit Care 2012;17(1):97–101.

91. Marcin J. Telemedicine in the pediatric intensive care unit. Pediatr Clin North Am 2013;60(3):581–90.

92. Vázquez de Anda FG, Rico SL, González Carbajal NP, et al. Medicina especializada presencial remota mediante el uso de robots en áreas críticas. Medicine Critica 2010;XXIV(4):178–84.

93. Petlin JB, Nelson ME, Goodman J. Deployment and early experience with remote-presence patient care in a community hospital. Surg Endosc 2007; 21(1):53–6.

94. Goran S. Measuring tele-ICU impact: does it optimize quality outcomes for the critically ill patient? J Nurs Manag 2012;20:414–28.

95. Rogove HJ, McArthur D, Demaerschalk BM, et al. Barriers to telemedicine: survey of current users in acute care units. Telemed J E Health 2012;18(1):48–53. http://dx.doi.org/10.1089/tmj.2011.0071.

96. Hulshoff L, Rood E, Cate J, et al. Telemedicine in the ICU, a review. Neth erlands J Crit Care 2011;15(1):9–12.

97. Cummings J, Krsek C, Vermoch K, et al. Intensive care unit telemedicine: review and consensus recommendations. Am J Med Qual 2007;22:239–50.

98. T-1 and T-3 line capability and cost. Available at: http://compnetworking.about.com/od/networkcables/f/t1_t3_lines.htm. Accessed July 18, 2014.

Index

Note: Page numbers of article titles are in **boldface** type.

Crit Care Clin 31 (2015) 351–377
http://dx.doi.org/10.1016/S0749-0704(15)00010-X
0749-0704/15/$ – see front matter © 2015 Elsevier Inc. All rights reserved.

Moving?

Make sure your subscription moves with you!

To notify us of your new address, find your **Clinics Account Number** (located on your mailing label above your name), and contact customer service at:

Email: journalscustomerservice-usa@elsevier.com

800-654-2452 (subscribers in the U.S. & Canada)
314-447-8871 (subscribers outside of the U.S. & Canada)

Fax number: 314-447-8029

Elsevier Health Sciences Division
Subscription Customer Service
3251 Riverport Lane
Maryland Heights, MO 63043

*To ensure uninterrupted delivery of your subscription, please notify us at least 4 weeks in advance of move.